Tongue Figure in Traditional Chinese Medicine

中医舌诊图谱

Tongue Figure In Traditional Chinese Medicine

中英文对照 (Chinese English)

主 编　丁成华
Chief Editor　Ding Chenghua
　　　　　孙晓刚
　　　　　Sun Xiaogang

人民卫生出版社
People's Medical Publishing House

编写人员

主编：
Editor-in-Chief：

丁成华（江西中医学院副教授、总策划）

Ding Chenghua（an associate professor in Jiang Xi college of traditional Chinese medicine，planner）

孙晓刚（南昌大学副教授、英译、英校）

Sun Xiaogang（an associate professor in Nan Chang University，the English reviser）

副主编：
Associate Editor-in-Chief：

黄丽萍（江西中医学院讲师、英译）

Huang Liping（lecturer in Jiang Xi college of traditional Chinese medicine，translator）

丁　明（南昌市第一医院副主任医师、资料收集与整理）

Ding Ming（an associate director in Nan Chang prot-hospital，collector and arranger of data）

马超英（江西中医学院教授、资料收集与整理）

Ma Chaoying（a professor in Jiang Xi college of traditional Chinese medicine，collector and arranger of data）

编委：（以姓氏笔画为序排列）
Editor-in-deputy：（in the order of the name of Chinese strokes in the surname）

丁成华（江西中医学院副教授、总策划）

Ding Chenghua（an associate professor in Jiang Xi college of traditional Chinese medicine，planner）

丁　明（南昌市第一医院副主任医师、资料收集与整理）

Ding Ming（an associate director in Nan Chang prot-hospital，collector and arranger of data）

马超英（江西中医学院教授、资料收集）

Ma Chaoying（a professor in Jiang Xi college of traditional Chinese medicine，collector and arranger of data）

孙晓刚（南昌大学副教授、英译、英校）

Sun Xiaogang (an associate professor in Nan Chang University, the English reviser)

乐毅敏(江西中医学院副教授、英校)
Le Yimin (an associate professor in Jiang Xi college of traditional Chinese medicine, the English reviser)

张　慧(江西中医学院实验师、摄像与图像处理)
Zhang Hui (an experimenter in JiangXi college of traditional Chinese medicine, photographer and image processor)

胡　珂(江西中医学院附属医院副主任医师、资料收集)
Hu Ke (an associate professor in JiangXi college of traditional Chinese medicine, collector of data)

陈耀辉(江西省人民医院主治医师、资料收集与整理)
Chen Yaohui (an attending physician in the People's Hospital of JiangXi Province, collector and arranger of data)

周志刚(江西中医学院助教、英译)
Zhou Zhigang (an teaching assistant in JiangXi college of traditional Chinese medicine, collector of data)

郭红飞(江西中医学院附属医院副主任医师、资料收集)
Guo Hongfei (an associate director in JiangXi college of traditional Chinese medicine, collector of data)

高秀娟(江西中医学院在读研究生,资料收集与整理)
Gao Xiujuan (a postgraduate in Jiang Xi college of traditional Chinese medicine, collector and arranger of data)

尚　姝(江西中医学院在读研究生,资料收集与整理)
Shang Shu (a postgraduate in Jiang Xi college of traditional Chinese medicine, collector and arranger of data)

汤希孟(江西中医学院教授、资料收集)
Tang XiMeng (a professor in Jiang Xi college of traditional Chinese medicine collector of data)

黄丽萍(江西中医学院讲师、英译)
Huang Liping (lecturer in Jiang Xi college of traditional Chinese medicine, translator)

章文春(江西中医学院副教授、资料收集与整理)
Zhang Wenchun (an associate professor in Jiang Xi college of traditional Chinese medicine, collector and arranger of data)

程海波(江西中医学院讲师,图像处理)
Cheng Haibo (lecturer in Jiang Xi college of traditional Chinese medicine, image processor)

前　言

舌诊是中医独具特色的诊断方法之一，为中医临床必察之项。古往今来，为名医者莫不精深于舌诊。

中医学认为，人体是一个有机的整体，舌象犹如反映人体生理病理的一面镜子。由于舌体与脏腑经络相连，舌络与气血津液相贯。故人体脏腑之虚实、气血之盛衰、津液之盈亏、胃气之存亡、病邪之性质、病情之轻重等信息均可通过舌诊而获得。

本书以中医理论为指导，充分吸取古今舌诊专著及此前各版中医诊断学教材与教参之精华。既全面继承中医舌诊之传统特色，又反映现代舌诊临床应用的最新成就。图文并茂、中英对照、内容翔实、文字精练、图像清晰、通俗易懂、科学实用是本书的一大特色。不仅扩大了读者范围，还为中医舌诊走向世界提供了宝贵的资源。

全书以绪论开篇，后分为四章论述。绪论中概述了中医舌诊的源流，介绍了古今舌诊专著；第一章为中医舌诊概要；第二章为诊舌质；第三章为诊舌苔；第四章为舌诊的临床意义及应用。本书采用高分辨率的数码相机，由摄影专业人员拍摄舌诊数字图像。编撰中精选了215幅高清晰度图像，将抽象的中医舌诊理论形象化、具体化，有助于读者学习、理解、掌握操作；有助于读者在头脑中形成并建立中医舌诊的诊断标准，从而促进中医舌诊的标准化、规范化。

舌诊内容虽多，舌象变化虽复杂，但总不离开舌质之神色形态与舌苔之苔质苔色的变化与组合。只要掌握了基本要领，就能执简驭繁，灵活应用，及时捕捉人体生理病理信息，做出准确诊断。

本书的读者对象与适用范围：

* 适合于全球中医药专业的本科生、研究生、留学生学习使用；
* 适合于中医、中西医结合的临床人员参考使用；
* 可作为医、教、研舌诊图像参考标准；
* 可供相关专业人员参考使用；
* 可供全球热爱中医、自学中医及重视自我保健者学习使用。

本书的出版，得到了江西省卫生厅的大力支持，在此表示衷心感谢！

编　者

2002.12.12

Preface

Tongue examination is one of unique exam method in traditional Chinese medicine (TCM). It is a necessary component in clinical diagnosis. Those famous doctor who lived in ancient society or live in modern society, are good at tongue-exam.

TCM considers the body of man is an inseparable whole and the tongue is just like a mirror that reflects physiological function and pathological changes. Because the tongue has closely related to viscera and qi, blood, and body fluid, the excess and deficiency of the visceral, the exuberance and decline of qi and blood, the wax and wane of body fluid, the existence and exhaustion of stomach qi, the nature of disease, and the deep and low location of disease, all can be reflected on the tongue.

Guided by theories of TCM, this book absorbs fully essentials from many monographs of tongue exam, and all kinds of editions of relevant all China TCM textbooks and reference books of higher learning. It not only inherits the traditional style of tongue exam, but also introduces the latest achievements of modern scientific research on tongue exam in TCM. Picture attached explanation, Chinese-English comparison, and sophisticated expression, clear picture writing manner and understandable language, science and practicality, all formes one of style of the book. Therefore, it not only widens the range of readers, but also supplies many valuable source of tongue exam to the world.

This book includes Introduction firstly and four chapters followed. The introduction mainly introduces the origin and development and monographs of tongue exam, the first chapter is covered with abstract of tongue exam, the second chapter includes observation of the tongue texture, third chapter reflects observation of the tongue clothing, the last chapter contents clinical significance and applications of tongue exam. In addition, professional photographer takes those pictures with a sophisticated machine. Over 200 pictures of tongue make the abstract theories of tongue exam concrete and imagery. That helps reader to understand the theories, master procedure and set a series of standards of tongue exam. It also promotes the process of setting up standard and regulation of tongue exam.

Although the contents of tongue exam is rich and the tongue picture is changeable and complex, it always varies in the range of tongue texture which includes tongue vitality, color, shape and movement, and tongue coating such as color and texture. If understand the basic method, we can seek some important information of disease, analyze the etiology and pathology, and summarize syndrome. So it's favorable to diagnose as soon as possible.

The book is suit for undergraduate, postgraduate and foreign students in medicinal college and university, especially for those who major Chinese Medicine and Pharmacology.

It's also suit for doctor who occupies TCM or combination of TCM with west Medicine (WM) in clinic.

Be used as the standard of tongue exam in clinic diagnosis, in field of teaching learning and in scientifically research.

Be utilized as a reference book for those whose major refers Chinese Medicine and Pharmacology.

Be suit for people who are interested in TCM, self-taught TCM and eager for keeping physique.

We have been greatly helped by the Health Department of Jiangxi Province during the publication of this book and we would like to express our profound thanks to them.

The Compiler
December. 12. 2002

目 录

绪论　Introduction …………………………………………………………………… 1
　1. 中医舌诊源流 ………………………………………………………………… 1
　1. The origin of the tongue inspection ………………………………………… 1
　2. 古今舌诊著作简介 …………………………………………………………… 5
　2. Brief introduction of tongue inspection monograph in ancient and
　　 modern times ………………………………………………………………… 5

第一章　舌诊概要 ………………………………………………………………… 14
Chapter one　Abstract …………………………………………………………… 14
　第一节　舌诊原理 ……………………………………………………………… 14
　Section 1　The Mechanism of Tongue Inspection ………………………… 14
　　1. 舌的形态结构和生理功能 ………………………………………………… 14
　　1. Structures and Physiological Function of Tongue ……………………… 14
　　　（1）形态结构 ……………………………………………………………… 14
　　　（1）Structures …………………………………………………………… 14
　　　（2）生理功能 ……………………………………………………………… 17
　　　（2）Function ……………………………………………………………… 17
　　2. 舌与脏腑经络、气血津液的关系 ………………………………………… 18
　　2. The Relationship Between Tongue and Viscera, Meridians Qi-$Blood$, and
　　　 Body Fluid ………………………………………………………………… 18
　　　（1）舌与脏腑经络的关系 ………………………………………………… 18
　　　（1）Tongue, Viscera and Meridians …………………………………… 18
　　　（2）舌与气血津液的关系 ………………………………………………… 20
　　　（2）The connection of tongue with, Qi, Blood and Body Fluid …… 20
　第二节　舌诊的方法与注意事项 ……………………………………………… 22
　Section 2　Method and Special attention on Observing Tongue ………… 22
　　1. 舌诊的基本操作 …………………………………………………………… 23
　　1. The Method of Tongue-Examination ……………………………………… 23
　　　（1）望舌的基本姿势 ……………………………………………………… 23
　　　（1）Posture ……………………………………………………………… 23
　　　（2）望舌的基本顺序 ……………………………………………………… 25

　　　　　(2) The Basic Procedure of Tongue-Observing ················ 25
　　　　(3) 舌诊的辅助手法 ················ 25
　　　　(3) Aiding Method of Tongue-observing ················ 25
　　　　　① 扣舌、摸舌 ················ 25
　　　　　① Toughing and Feeling ················ 25
　　　　　② 揩舌、刮舌 ················ 26
　　　　　② Scrubbing and Scraping ················ 26
　　2. 舌诊的注意事项 ················ 28
　　2. Special Attentions on observing Tongue ················ 28
　　　　(1) 光线条件 ················ 29
　　　　(1) Light ················ 29
　　　　(2) 食物或药品影响 ················ 29
　　　　(2) Diet and Drugs ················ 29
　　　　(3) 口腔对舌象的影响 ················ 31
　　　　(3) Effect of Buccal Cavity ················ 31
　第三节　舌诊的基本内容和正常舌象 ················ 32
　Section 3　Content of Tongue Inspection and Normal Tongue ················ 32
　　1. 舌诊的基本内容 ················ 32
　　1. Contents of Tongue Inspection ················ 32
　　2. 正常舌象 ················ 33
　　2. The Normal Tongue Picture ················ 33
　　3. 舌象的生理变异 ················ 34
　　3. Physiological change of Tongue ················ 34
　　　　(1) 年龄、性别因素 ················ 34
　　　　(1) Age and Sex ················ 34
　　　　(2) 体质禀赋因素 ················ 36
　　　　(2) Constitution and Congenital Disposition ················ 36
　　　　(3) 气候环境因素 ················ 37
　　　　(3) Climate and Environment ················ 37
　　　　(4) 生活起居习性因素 ················ 38
　　　　(4) Habits and Customs ················ 38

第二章　诊舌质 ················ 42
Chapter Two Observation of the tongue texture ················ 42
　第一节　诊舌神 ················ 42
　Section 1　Observations of the tongue vitality ················ 42
　　1. 有神 ················ 42
　　1. Full vitality ················ 42
　　2. 无神 ················ 43

  2. Lacking of vitality (out of vitality) ·· 43
 第二节 诊舌色 ·· 44
 Section Two Observations of The Tongue Color ·································· 44
  1. 淡红舌 ·· 44
  1. The Pink Tongue ·· 44
  2. 淡白舌 ·· 44
  2. The Pale Tongue ·· 44
  3. 红舌 ·· 46
  3. The Red Tongue ·· 46
  4. 绛舌 ·· 49
  4. The Crimson Tongue ·· 49
  5. 紫舌 ·· 50
  5. The Purple Tongue ··· 50
  6. 青舌 ·· 52
  6. The Blue Tongue ·· 52
 第三节 诊舌形 ·· 53
 Section 3 Observation of the Tongue Shape ····································· 53
  1. 苍老舌 ·· 53
  1. The Tough Tongue ··· 53
  2. 娇嫩舌 ·· 53
  2. The Tender Tongue ··· 53
  3. 胖大舌 ·· 54
  3. The Swelling Tongue ·· 54
  4. 瘦薄舌 ·· 56
  4. The Thin Tongue ··· 56
  5. 点、刺舌 ·· 57
  5. The Spotted or Prickled Tongue ··· 57
  6. 裂纹舌 ·· 59
  6. The Fissured Tongue ··· 59
  7. 齿痕舌 ·· 61
  7. The Teeth Printed Tongue ··· 61
 第四节 诊舌态 ·· 62
 Section 4 Observation of The Moving State of The Tongue ················ 62
  1. 痿软舌 ·· 62
  1. The Flaccid Tongue ·· 62
  2. 强硬舌 ·· 63
  2. The Stiff Tongue ··· 63
  3. 歪斜舌 ·· 65
  3. The Wry Tongue ··· 65

4. 颤动舌 ··· 66

　　4. The Trembling Tongue ··· 66

　　5. 吐弄舌 ··· 67

　　5. The Protruding And Licking Tongue ·· 67

　　6. 短缩舌 ··· 68

　　6. The Shortened Tongue ··· 68

　第五节　诊舌下络脉 ·· 69

　Section 5　Observations of The Vessels Below Tongue ····································· 69

　　1. 舌下络脉的观察方法 ··· 70

　　1. Methods of Observing The Vessels Below Tongue ···································· 70

　　2. 舌下络脉异常及其临床意义 ·· 70

　　2. The Clinical Significance of Abnormal Hypoglossal Vessels ······················· 70

第三章　诊舌苔 ·· 72
Chapter 3 Observations of The Tongue Coating ·· 72

　第一节　诊苔质 ··· 73

　Section 1 Observations of The Texture of Tongue Coating ··································· 73

　　1. 薄苔、厚苔 ··· 73

　　1. Thickness and Thinness ··· 73

　　2. 润苔、燥苔 ··· 77

　　2. Moistness and Dryness ·· 77

　　3. 腻苔、腐苔 ··· 81

　　3. Putrid and Greasiness ·· 81

　　4. 剥苔 ·· 84

　　4. Exfoliation ·· 84

　　5. 偏苔、全苔 ··· 87

　　5. Evenness and Unevenness ··· 87

　　6. 真苔、假苔 ··· 89

　　6. The True and False Coating ·· 89

　第二节　诊苔色 ··· 90

　Section 2 Color of Tongue Coating ·· 90

　　1. 白苔 ·· 91

　　1. White Coating ··· 91

　　2. 黄苔 ·· 93

　　2. The Yellow Coating ·· 93

　　3. 灰苔、黑苔 ··· 97

　　3. The Gray and Black Coating ··· 97

第四章　舌诊的临床意义及应用 ·· 100

Chapter 4 The Usage and Significance of Tongue Inspection ………………… 100
  第一节　舌诊的临床意义 ………………………………………………………… 100
  Section 1 Significance of Tongue Inspection ……………………………………… 100
    1. 判断邪正盛衰 ……………………………………………………………………… 101
    1. To judge the exuberance or decline of the *vital-qi* **and the** *pathogenic-qi* …… 101
    2. 区别病邪性质 ……………………………………………………………………… 101
    2. To distinguish the nature of disease ………………………………………… 101
    3. 判别病位浅深 ……………………………………………………………………… 102
    3. To detect the shallow or deep location of disease ………………………… 102
    4. 推断病势进退 ……………………………………………………………………… 103
    4. To infer the Tendency of disease ……………………………………………… 103
    5. 估计病情预后 ……………………………………………………………………… 103
    5. To Estimate the Prognosis of Disease ………………………………………… 103
  第二节　舌诊的临床应用 ………………………………………………………… 104
  Section 2 Clinical Application of Tongue Inspection …………………………… 104
    1. 舌诊在温病诊治中的应用 ………………………………………………………… 104
    1. Application of tongue inspection in diagnosing and treating febrile disease … 104
      （1）辨舌苔探病邪性质、病位浅深 ………………………………………… 104
      （1）To judge the nature of disease and to detect the location of disease …… 104
      （2）辨舌色定卫气营血、病情轻重 ………………………………………… 105
      （2）To judge Wei-qi-yin-xue and the condition of disease ………………… 105
    2. 舌诊在心血管疾病诊治中的应用 ………………………………………………… 106
    2. Application of tongue inspection in diagnosing and treating cardiovascular disease …………………………………………………………………………… 106
      （1）心肌梗死 …………………………………………………………………… 106
      （1）Myocardial infarction ……………………………………………………… 106
      （2）冠心病心绞痛 ……………………………………………………………… 108
      （2）Angina pectoris …………………………………………………………… 108
      （3）房颤 ………………………………………………………………………… 108
      （3）Atrial fibrillation …………………………………………………………… 108
    3. 舌诊在肺系疾病诊治中的应用 …………………………………………………… 109
    3. Application of tongue inspection in diagnosing and treating lung disease …… 109
      （1）慢性支气管炎、肺心病 ………………………………………………… 109
      （1）Chronic bronchitis, pulmonary heart disease …………………………… 109
      （2）肺癌 ………………………………………………………………………… 110
      （2）Lung cancer ………………………………………………………………… 110
    4. 舌诊在脾胃疾病诊治中的应用 …………………………………………………… 110
    4. Application of tongue inspection in diagnosing and treating spleen and stomach disease …………………………………………………………………… 110

　　　　(1) 慢性胃炎 ·· 111
　　　　(1) Chronic gastritis ··· 111
　　　　(2) 胃及十二指肠溃疡 ······································· 111
　　　　(2) Gastric ulcer and duodenalulcer ························ 111
　　　　(3) 急性阑尾炎 ·· 112
　　　　(3) Acute appendicitis ······································· 112
　　5．舌诊在肝胆疾病诊治中的应用 ································ 113
　　5．Application of tongue inspection in diagnosing and treating liver and
　　　gallbladder disease ··· 113
　　　　(1) 乙型肝炎及肝癌 ··· 113
　　　　(1) B hepatitis and liver cancer ······························ 113
　　　　(2) 胆囊炎、胆结石 ··· 114
　　　　(2) Cholecystitis，Cholelithiasis ···························· 114
　　6．舌诊在肾脏疾病诊治中的应用 ································ 115
　　6．Application of tongue inspection in diagnosing and treating kidney disease
　　　 ··· 115
　　7．舌诊在内分泌疾病诊治中的应用 ······························ 116
　　7．Application of tongue in diagnosing and treating endocrinopathy ········ 116

参考文献 ·· 118
Reference documents ·· 118

绪 论

Introduction

舌诊是通过观察病人舌质和舌苔的变化,以诊察疾病的方法。舌诊具有悠久的历史,早在《黄帝内经》中就有望舌诊病的记载,经历代医家对舌诊理论研究和临床应用,使舌诊理论体系和诊断方法不断发展,日臻完善。

Tongue inspection is a method to diagnose the disease by inspecting the patient's change of the tongue texture and the tongue coating. Tongue inspection has a long history, and was recorded as early as in the *Huang di Internal Medicine*, the tongue inspection and the diagnostic method has been continuously developed and got consummated through research on the tongue inspection and the clinic applications by successive dynasties doctors.

1. 中医舌诊源流
1. The origin of the tongue inspection

中医舌诊历史悠久,早在殷墟甲骨文中就有"贞疾舌"的记载。贞者,占也,验也。是对舌病与验舌的最早记载。

Tongue inspection on the traditional Chinese Medicine has a long history, early in the Yin dynasty it was recorded by Chinese inscription on bones and tortoise shells that "zhen can diagnose the tongue disease". zhen, meaning divine or effectiveness, and is the earliest record for tongue disease and inspecting tongue.

战国时期,扁鹊(秦越人)即以切脉、望色、听声、写形等多种诊法诊病。扁鹊舌诊的内容,曾被《脉经》所辑录,其中有舌诊四则。如《脉经》转录的《扁鹊诊诸反逆死脉要诀》第五中有"偏枯……不喑舌转,可治,"的记载。指出偏枯,不能说话而舌体能转动者,为轻证,较易治愈。是据舌体转动灵活的程度,对中风偏枯做出诊断和预后。扁鹊舌诊的内容虽仅4条,但论述十分精辟,为后世舌诊奠定了基础。

During Zhanguo period, Bian que or QinYueren, diagnosed disease by pulse, observation, auscultation and observing the constitution. The contents of Bian que's tongue inspection was compiled in the *Pulse classic* in which recorded four tongue inspection, for example, *The Fifth Key Point for All The Dying Pulse* which was compiled in *Pulse Classic* said "withering tongue… If the voice is not aphonic and the tongue can turn, the patients can be cured,". It pointed out that a withering tongue, which could turn but not speak was a slight syndrome and could be cured. According to the extent of the tongue movement, the doctors can make diagnosis and prognosis. Although the contents of the Bian que's diagnosis were only four, the statements were very penetrating, which had laid a foundation for tongue inspection for latter generations.

《黄帝内经》成书的战国时期,舌诊的运用已占一定地位。《内经》对舌的解剖、功能、舌与内脏,经脉的关系,舌诊的临床应用等,均有论述。《灵枢·经脉》说:"唇舌者,肌肉之本也。脉不荣则肌肉软,肌肉软则舌萎。"指明舌体是以肌肉为主构成的器官,受血脉的充养,舌失荣养即痿软不用。《灵枢·五阅五使》说:"舌者,心之官也。"舌的功能与形态的变异,不仅能反映心的病变,也能反映其他脏腑的病变。在《灵枢·经脉》中记载了五脏六腑皆通过经脉直接或间接与舌相通。脏腑之经脉通于舌,脏腑功能及气血津液的病变也必然反映于舌。故察舌的形态、色泽、润燥、口味等变异,可以诊断脏腑、气血、津液的病变,这是《内经》对舌诊机制的基本认识。

Tongue inspection has had a important role in Zhanguo dynasty when *Huang Di Internal Classic* was formed. *Internal Classic* has made statements about the tongue anatomy, function, relationship with viscera collaterals, meridians and clinical application of tongue inspection. *Spirit Pivot* said "lip and tongue are the material base of the muscle, the pulses which are not nourished can led to soft muscle, the soft muscle can result in atrophy of the tongue." That is to say that the body of tongue is a organ mainly made up of muscle. The tongue failing to be nourished can lead to atrophy and softness. *Spirit Pivot* said "the tongue is a organ of the heart". The changes of the functions and shapes of tongue can not only reflect the heart disease, but the pathogenic changes of other zang and fu viscera. *Spirit Pivot* said that the five-zang and six-fu viscera pass through the tongue directly or indirectly through the meridians and collaterals. The meridians and collaterals of zang and fu viscera connect with the tongue, so the functions of zang and fu viscera and changes of the qi, blood and body fluid could be inevitably manifested on the tongue. Therefore by observing the changes of shapes, color, dryness moistness and taste, we can diagnose the pathogenic changes of zang and fu viscera, qi, blood and body fluid, these are the basic principles of the tongue inspection's mechanism in *Internal Classic*.

自《内经》以降,经历代医家对舌诊的不断探索,其理论日趋完备。东汉张仲景《伤寒杂病论》载舌诊内容20余条,并提出了"舌胎"一词,张石顽《伤寒绪论》释曰:"舌胎之名,始于长沙,以其邪气传里,如有所怀,故谓之胎。"后人将舌上苔垢称为"舌苔",并沿用至今。"邪中与脏,舌即难言",确立舌诊作为辨证论治的依据。晋·王叔和《脉经》虽为脉诊专著,但书中也不乏以舌诊佐脉诊病的例证,表明晋代已发展了《伤寒杂病论》舌脉互参的诊病方法。

From *Internal Classic* on, the theory of tongue inspection gradually becomes perfection through continually exploration on tongue inspection by doctors in successive dynasties. Zhang Zhongjing, the famous doctor in Donghan dynasty, proposed a new word "tongue coating" in his works *Treatise on Cold-Attack* which recorded about more than 20 contents of tongue inspection. Zhang Shiwan explained it in *Introduction of Treatise on Cold-Attack* "the name of tongue coating, is originated from changshan. Because the evils transmit interior, just like pregnancy, so it was called tongue coating". the latter doctors called the fur-like material "tongue coating". And lasted till now. Wang Shuhe, the famous doctor in Jing dynasty, recorded a lot of cases about the tongue inspection helping diagnose diseases in his works *Pulse Classic* which is a monograph about tongue inspection, all these indicate that Jing dynasty had developed a diagnostic method combining *Treatise on Cold-Attack* with tongue inspection.

隋·巢元方《诸病源候论》提出了舌强、舌缩、舌胀、舌不收、舌燥、舌烂、重舌、舌上生疮、舌上白、舌上黄、舌上白黄、舌焦黑、舌赤、舌青、舌赤黑、舌上胎滑等多种舌象及其临床意义,在舌诊研究与运用上,较《伤寒杂病论》进了一大步。

In Sui dynasty, Chao Yuanfang proposed in his works *The General Treatise on The Causes And Symptoms of Diseases* the clinical significance of tongue inspection and tongue picture, such as tongue stiffness, tongue shortness, tongue corpulence, protruding tongue, tongue dryness, tongue ulcer, double tongue, tongue carbuncle, yellow tongue, white tongue, yellow and white tongue, dark-black tongue, red tongue, blue tongue, dark-red tongue and slippery tongue. It has made a great progress than that of *Treatise on Cold-Attack* on the researches and applications of tongue inspection.

唐·孙思邈《千金方》卷14〈舌论〉为中医专论舌诊之发端。宋、金时期,《活人书》以有无口燥舌干来辨阴阳虚实,《小儿药证直诀》首创"舒舌"、"弄舌"的名称。以上文献中所记载舌诊的内容丰富,但比较分散,只是舌诊学的雏形,还不能算是舌诊学的专著。

In Tang dynasty, *A Thousand Gold Worthy Prescription* compiled by Sun simiao is the beginning of tongue inspection monograph. During the Jing, Song dynasties, *Books on Surviving Patients* differentiated yin, yang, deficiency, excess on the basis of having dry mouth or not, *Key to Therapeutics of Children's Disease* firstly proposed "extended tongue" "licking tongue". All the documents mentioned above were abundant in contents but scattered, which is only an embryonic form, not a real monograph of tongue inspection.

元代《敖氏金镜录》总结了12舌图为中医舌论第一专著。这也是世界上最早的舌诊专书。后经同代人杜清碧增至36舌图,因下列治则方药,使此书更加完善,被后人称为《敖氏伤寒金镜录》而成为舌诊的开山之作。《金镜录》认为,诊舌可以起到"推摊寻流,实可决死生之妙"的作用。该书以图文两种形式撰成,成为继《内经》、《伤寒论》、《诸病源候论》、《千金方》之后,集元代舌诊之大成的舌诊力作,该书对舌苔进退发展规律之精辟论断,一直沿用至今。

Ao's Golden Mirror compiled in Yuan dynasty is the earliest existing monograph on tongue inspection, and is earliest existing monograph in the world, which summed up 12 tongue pictures. Du Qingbi, same generation of Ao's, increased the tongue picture by 36, And below the tongue picture, Du listed the therapeutic principle and formula, making this book more perfect. This works is called *Ao's Golden Mirror of Cold-Attack Disease* by the latter people, and becomes the founder of a religious sect of tongue inspection. *Ao's Golden Mirror of Cold-Attack Disease* considered that tongue inspection has functions of "distinguishing the live from death", After *Internal Medicine*, *Treatise on Cold-Attack*, *The General Treatise on The Causes And Symptoms of Diseases*, *A Thousand Gold Worthy Prescriptions*, this book was compiled in two forms summed up the great achievements of tongue inspection in Yuan dynasty, and was regarded as a monumental work. The penetrating statements on the role of disease tendency lasted till now.

明清两代研究舌诊者日增,使舌诊研究进入了一个新阶段。舌诊专著不断涌现,实用性较强。明清两代的温病学派,对诊舌辨证做了大量探索。吴又可、叶天士、薛生白、吴鞠通、王孟英等人,都极重视舌诊在诊断温病中的重要作用,并在各自的著作中丰富了温病辨证的舌论理论。

More and more tongue researchers during the Ming dynasty and Qing dynasty have taken the tongue research step into a new stage. A lot of tongue inspection monograph which had comparative practical use announced to come into being. The school of seasonal febrile disease in the period of the Ming dynasty and Qing dynasty has made enormous explorations. For example, Wu Youke, Ye Tianshi, Xue Shengbai, Wu Jutong, Wang Mengying etc, extremely emphasized the important role of tongue inspection in diagnosing the seasonal febrile disease, and enriched the tongue inspection theory of the differentiation of the seasonal febrile disease in their works respectively.

建国后,舌诊研究进入了快速发展的新阶段。重新整理出版了前人医著中临床实用价值较大的舌诊医籍,利用各种现代科学手段研究舌诊,舌诊在临床诊治疾病中得到广泛应用,并取得了许多可喜的研究成果。丰富了中医舌诊理论,提高了舌诊的临床实用价值。

After the foundation of the People's Republic of china, the tongue inspection researches have stepped into a rapidly developing new stage. A lot of ancient medical works after rearrangement were published. The modern researchers have made best use of all modern scientific methods to research tongue inspection and made great achievements, tongue inspection was widely applied in diagnosing and treating disease, Which enriched the tongue inspection theory and improved the clinically practical value.

2. 古今舌诊著作简介
2. Brief introduction of tongue inspection monograph in ancient and modern times

(1)《敖氏伤寒金镜录》又名《伤寒舌诊》,元·杜本(清碧)撰于 1341 年现存光绪年间上海锦章书局石印本。此书原书仅有舌苔图谱 12 幅,后经杜清碧根据其本人的临床经验整理又增加 24 图,合成 36 舌图,并在图下列出治则与方药,使其更趋完善。此书是我国第一部整理研究舌诊的专著,它的问世标志着我国舌诊研究至元代已成为一个研究专题,从而使舌诊研究进入了一个新的发展阶段。

(1) *Ao's Golden Mirror of Cold-Attack Disease*, also called *Tongue Inspection on Cold-Attack Disease*, was compiled in 1341, and published by the shanghai Jinzhang publishing house. The original works only had 12 pictures of tongue coating. Latter Du qingbi added 24 pictures of tongue coating after his rearrangement according to his own clinic experiences, so the pictures of this works are 36. Below the tongue picture, Du listed the therapeutic principle and formula, making this book comparative perfection. This works is the earliest monograph which was rearranged to research the tongue inspection. *Ao's Golden Mirror of Cold-Attack Disease* marked that tongue inspection research in Yuan dynasty has been a monographic study which made tongue inspection research step into a newly developing stage.

(2)《伤寒观舌心法》明·申斗垣(拱辰)撰。此书是在《敖氏伤寒金镜录》36 舌图的基础上,演绎为 137 舌,其内容丰富,阐述精辟,是申氏多年来临床实践的总结,集当时舌诊之大成,是为一代名著。

(2) *The Experience of Tongue Observation on The Cold-Attack Disease* was written by Shen douyuan in Ming dynasty. the tongue pictures in this works were deduced to 137 tongue pictures on the basis of *Ao's Golden Mirror of Cold-Attack Disease*. Its contents are abundant and the statements are penetrating. It was clinically practical summary of Dou's, and summed up great achievements of tongue inspection of that time, so it is a famous works.

(3)《伤寒舌鉴》清·张登(诞先)撰于 1668 年。此书取《观舌心法》之精华,正其误错,去其繁芜。此书备列《伤寒观舌之法》,分白、黑、黄、灰、红、紫、酱、蓝等 8 种舌苔,共成 120 舌苔图。并附妊娠伤寒舌,每种舌除总论之外,各图均有说明,观舌辨证,颇为扼要;该书首次将望舌分出苔、质,阐述了前人未有之望舌经验。

(3) *Differentiation of The Tongue Pictures on The Cold-Attack Disease* was written by Zhang Deng in 1668, this works was on basis of *The Experience of Tongue Observation*, but Zhang selected the finest, corrected the mistakes, removed the errors and the verbose, completely listed the methods of observing tongue, so there were 120 tongue pictures in his works, this works listed completely the methods of tongue in-

spection, and divided 8 tongue coating categories such as white, black, yellow, gray, red, purple, dark reddish brown, blue and having a appendix on cold-attack tongue in pregnant woman. Except for the introduction, every picture had indications, observing tongue and differentiation is brief and to the point. In this book the tongue observation firstly divided into tongue coating, tongue texture and elaborated the experiences which the previous doctor had never elaborated before.

(4)《舌鉴总论》清·徐大椿(灵胎)撰于1764年。此书舌诊内容大部分摘录张登的《伤寒舌鉴》,个人的经验并不多,但对于舌白、舌黄、舌黑、舌红、舌紫、舌蓝等舌的归纳,文字精当,亦有可取之处。

(4) *Introduction of The Tongue Differentiation* was written by Xu Lingtai in 1764 in which his own experience were not enough, most of tongue inspection contents were abstracted from *Differentiation of The Tongue Pictures on The Cold-Attack Disease*, but the conclusions on white coating, yellow coating, black coating, red coating, purple coating and blue coating were penetrating and worthy reference.

(5)《伤寒舌鉴》清·王文选撰于1838年,载于清·刘以仁所著的《活人心法》卷中部分(1902年)。该书集杜本36舌、张登120舌、段正谊《瘟疫论》13舌,择录其中149舌而成。此书对温热病辨舌经验较以前有不少补充,且有特色,为清代以前舌诊学之总汇。

(5) *Differentiation of The Tongue Pictures on The Cold-Attack Disease* was written by Wang Wenxuan in 1838, and compiled in parts of *The Experience of Surviving Patients* (1902). This book summed up 36 tongue pictures in Du's works, 120 tongue pictures in Zhang Deng's works, 13 tongue pictures in Duang Zhengyi's works (*Treatise on Pestilence*), and selected 149 tongue pictures of them. In this book, the experiences about tongue differentiation on seasonal febrile disease supplemented much more than before, and had characteristic feature and was a summary of tongue inspection before Qing dynasty.

(6)《舌胎统志》清·傅松元(耐寒)撰于1874年。此书一改古代医家以苔色分门而从舌色分类。全书将舌色分为枯白舌、淡白舌、淡红舌、正红舌、绛舌、紫舌、青舌、黑舌等8种舌色,其内容丰富,颇多经验之谈,其中尤以淡白舌、枯白舌的病理描述最为精当;淡白舌一名,也由傅氏在该书中首创,以有别于淡红舌。

(6) *The General Records of The Tongue and Coating* was written by Fu Songyuan in 1874, the category of tongue color differentiated from the category of coating color by other doctors, This works divided the tongue color into 8 tongue color such as withering white tongue, pale tongue, reddish tongue, red tongue, crimson tongue, purplish tongue, blue tongue, black tongue. There were abundant in contents and a lot of clinical experiences in this book. The pathogenic descriptions on pale tongue and withering tongue were very precise, The name of pale tongue which was different from the reddish

tongue, firstly created by him.

(7)《舌鉴辨正》清·梁玉瑜(特岩)撰于1894年。该书是取王文选《舌鉴》为原本,逐条辨其谬误,正其偏差,并增入杂病观舌辨证之法而成。该书强调"分经辨证"察舌,重视"刮舌验苔",不但辨其外感,且兼辨内伤。由于该书敢于辨谬纠偏,实事求是,是一本对我国舌诊学有重要贡献的参考书。

(7) *The Correctness of Differentiation of Tongue* was written by Liang Yushu in 1894, this book was originated from the *Differentiation of Tongue* written by Wang Wenxian, it corrected the mistakes step by step, what's more, added the differentiation of syndrome by observing tongue for miscellaneous diseases. Liang emphasized to observe the tongue according to meridian syndrome differentiation, and attached importance to "examining the coating by scraping the tongue". The author not only differentiated the exogenous evil attacking diseases but also the miscellaneous diseases. This book contributed lots to tongue inspection in China because the author dared to distinguish errors and to correct mistakes and to seek the truth from facts

(8)《察舌辨证新法》清·刘恒瑞撰写于1911年。作者继承祖国医学传统辨舌经验,结合一些现代医学知识写成是书。该书主要论述白、黄、黑三种舌苔的诊察方法,并论及辨舌苔变化以测吉凶和舌苔的真假消退等,均有所创见。全书叙述明了,理论结合实际,诊断与治法并提,颇能指导临床。

(8) *New Differentiation of Syndrome by Observing Tongue* was written by Liu Hengrui in 1911, The author combined the traditional experiences of differentiating tongue with modern medicine knowledge. This book mainly stated 3 examining methods of observing white, yellow, black tongue and coating, and involved in differentiating the changes of tongue and to make a prognosis, also to including the wax and wane, false and true of tongue coating. All the ideas' of author's mentioned above were creative. These works were stated precisely and simply, and could guide the clinic because of its integration of theory and practice and combination diagnosis with therapeutic principles.

(9)《辨舌指南》民国·曹炳章(赤电)撰于1917年。曹氏以其精湛的医术,博学多识之才,广采古今各家医书156家,国内外近译医书30余部及各报杂志30余种,凡察舌治病之法,摘录无遗,并去繁就简,去粕存精,写成有彩图122幅,黑白图6幅的舌诊类书名著。由于该书力集古人舌诊经验于一全,并能初步运用现代医学解剖、组织、生理学观点来阐明中医舌诊原理,如舌之大体解剖和一些细微结构(舌乳头、味蕾、血管、神经),此书内容充实,是我国舌诊学清以前集大成者,是研究舌诊的重要著作。

(9) *A Guide to Differentiate The Tongue And Coating* was written by Cao Bingzhang in 1917, Cao completed this works by his consummately medical skills, learned and versatile talent because he numerously collected 156 kinds of medical books from ancient period to modern period and about more than 30 recently translated medical

books and all kinds of newspapers and magazines. This book included all the methods of differentiating tongue and treating diseases and discarded the dross and selected the essential. This book is a famous encyclopedia including 122 colorful tongue picture and 6 black-and-white tongue picture. As it contributed to sum up all the experiences of ancient doctors in one book and could firstly apply the modern anatomy, histology, physiology knowledge which he used to expound the mechanism of tongue inspection, for example, the anatomy of the tongue body and substructure (lingual papillae, gustatory bud, vessels, nerves). This works is abundant in contents and a famous works for research which summed up great achievements prior to Qing dynasty.

(10)《临症验舌法》民国·杨云峰撰写于1923年。全书分上、下两卷。上卷总论，以舌、苔的形态、颜色分析病情的虚实阴阳，验舌以分脏腑，并密切结合治法，每种舌象均配以主方；下卷方论，介绍各方的适用证和用法。该书提出的《辨舌分配脏腑法》、《验舌分虚实法》、《验舌分阴阳法》为后来舌诊研究提供了重要参考。由于作者企图由博返约，化繁为简，因而对中医舌诊学渊博之学问不能尽言，使该书实成为舌诊学中的简书而已。

(10) *Examining Tongue Methods for Medical Practice* divided into 2 volumes, was written by Yang Yunfeng in 1923. The first volume which was an introduction analyzed the pathogenic conditions of excess and deficiency and Yin and Yang by texture and color of the tongue and coating, differentiated zang-fu viscera by examining tongue, listed the main formula for every tongue picture closely relating the therapeutic principles; The second volume was a statement about formulas which introduced the indications and directions. *Differentiating Zang and Fu Viscera According to Tongue*, *Differentiation of Tongue According to Excess And Deficiency*, *Differentiation of Tongue According to Yin Yang* proposed by Yang afforded a important reference for the latter researchers. The author intended to make the tongue inspection precisely and appropriately, so he couldn't expound in details for the broad and profound tongue inspection, therefore this works was a simple book elaborating tongue inspection.

(11)《国医舌诊学》民国·邱骏声撰写于1933年。该书有系统地整理了中医舌诊的有关文献，其内容丰富，颇有体会，且条分缕析，很是醒目。全书分上、中、下三篇，上篇分述舌诊学之定义、历史、范围、价值，舌体生理构造、功能和内应脏腑部位；中篇除察舌辨证纲要外，分述苔色、苔质、舌色、舌体、味觉辨证方法和舌诊特殊状态；下篇为舌诊图解，结合方药，阐述了145种不同舌图的辨证论治。

(11) *Tongue Inspection of Motherland Medicine* was written by Qiu Junsheng in 1933. This eye-catching book systematically arranged relevant documents on tongue inspection and was abundant in content with plenty of experiences, the author explained statements in details. This book was divided into three volumes, in which the first volume elaborated the definition, history, scope, value of tongue inspection, physiological structure and functions of the tongue body and the portions corresponding with internal

Zang and Fu viscera;The second volume expounded the coating color ,tongue texture ,tongue color ,tongue body ,differentiation of taste sense and special status of tongue inspection ;The third volume which was a picture explanation of tongue inspection elaborated 145 differentiation of tongue according to different tongue picture

(12)《中医舌诊》北京中医学院中医系中医基础理论教研组编,人民卫生出版社1960年7月出版。这是建国后的第一本舌诊专著,简述了舌诊发展史、舌的构造及与脏腑的关系、舌诊的临床意义、舌苔的诊察方法和舌质的诊察,并重点介绍了临床常见各种舌质结合舌苔的主病和治法。此书继承了祖国医学的舌诊学实质和精华,并有所发挥和进展。此书叙述简明,深入浅出,内容广博而不杂乱,是一本优秀的舌诊参考书籍,对我国舌诊研究和教学都产生了深远的影响。

(12) *Tongue Inspection in Traditional Chinese Medicine* , published by people's hygiene publishing house in 1960, was compiled by basic T.C.M theory teaching and research group of T.C.M department in Beijing institution of T.C.M. This was the first monograph of tongue inspection after the people's republic of china was founded , It not only briefly introduced the history of tongue inspection、structure of tongue and its relationship with zang and fu viscera ,clinic significance of tongue inspection,examining methods of tongue coating and examination of the tongue texture ,but also emphatically introduced kinds of tongue textures combined with the indications and therapeutic principles often seen in clinic practice. The authors inherited the essence of tongue inspection and made plenty of development and great progress. This book stated briefly, explained the profound in simple terms, and its contents were broad but not mixed and disorderly, so it was a excellent reference book and gave rise to a profound influence on the latter researches and teaching.

(13)《舌诊研究》陈泽霖、陈梅芳编著,上海科学技术出版社1965年出版,1982年再版。该书系中西医结合研究舌诊的专著。作者运用现代解剖、组胚、生理、生化、病理等方法研究舌诊,中西医结合,融会贯通。该书叙述了舌诊的发展概况、临床意义和诊察方法;详述已有的各种舌诊研究方法;正常舌象和病理舌象,每种舌象都附有临床实例,分析出该舌象形成的有关因子,并提出了作者的独创性看法。作者结合临床经验,对每种病理舌象概括性地提出了临床辨证类型,对临床察舌辨证也有一定的指导意义。

(13) *The Researches of Tongue Inspection* , published by Shanghai Scientific Technology Publishing House in 1965,was compiled by Chen Zelin and Chen Meifang , and republished in 1982 after being revised . It was a monograph on tongue inspection combining T.C.M with west medicine. Authors applied the modern anatomy, histology and embryology, biology and chemistry, physiology, pathology , pathological physiology to research the tongue inspection ,and gained a thorough understanding of tongue inspection through mastery of all relevant material with a method by combining T.C.M with western medicine. This book narrated the general condition of developments , clinical

significance and methods of tongue observation; and elaborated all kinds of research methods of tongue inspection、normal tongue pictures and pathogenic tongue pictures below which the authors attached clinic cases; And analyzed the relevant factors about the formation of tongue,what's more, they proposed their own creative ideas, and drew a summary conclusions on clinic differentiation for every pathogenic tongue which could guide the clinic differentiation of tongue inspection.

(14)《中医舌苔图谱》宋天彬编著,人民卫生出版社1984年9月出版。此书共有彩图舌象257幅,是当时我国舌诊研究彩图篇幅较多的图谱。全书重点介绍了舌诊的原理、临床意义、舌质与舌苔的关系、舌诊方法与注意事项和舌诊内容五部分;图谱部分包括正常舌类、淡白舌类、淡红舌类、红舌类、绛舌类、青紫舌类和其他舌类七部分。该书是一部形象直观、突出了单因素的临床意义的舌诊图谱专著。

(14) *Atlas of Tongue Coating of T.C.M*, published by the People's Hygiene Publishing House in September, 1984, was compiled by Song Tianbin. This book contained 257 colorful photos of tongue picture, which had comparatively more photos than those of previous books of that time. The author emphatically introduced the principles of tongue inspection, clinic significance, relationship between tongue texture and tongue coating, methods on tongue inspection and cautions and five parts of tongue inspection. The atlas part was divided into 7 parts such as normal tongue category, pale tongue part, reddish tongue part, red tongue part, crimson tongue part, blue and purplish tongue parts and other part. So this work was a directly perceived tongue atlas which stressed single-factor clinic significance.

(15)《望舌诊病》李乃民著,黑龙江科学技术出版社1987年3月出版。此书特点是在中医察舌辨证的基础上,结合现代医学手段和临床经验,首次提出了望舌与现代医学的单一疾病相联系的望舌诊病方法,作者总结了内科、外科、妇科24种疾病舌象的表征,使舌象第一次在舌诊专著中成为对某一疾病的诊断标准。

(15) *Diagnosing Diseases by Inspecting Tongue*, published by Heilongjiang Scientific Technology Publishing House in March ,1987, was written by Li Naimin. The character of this book was the first one to propose a method to diagnose diseases by tongue inspection combining tongue inspection with a single disease in modern medicine on the basis of differentiation of tongue inspection combining modern technology with clinic experience. The author summed up 24 tongue symbols of internal medicine disease, surgical disease and gynecological diseases and it was the first time to make the tongue picture as diagnostic standard of a certain disease.

(16)《中国舌诊大全》李乃民主编,学苑出版社1994年2月出版。全书分上、中、下三篇。上篇为中国古医籍舌诊,对先秦、西汉至1949年间的舌诊医籍作了系统的整理研究;中篇为建国后舌诊及非舌诊专著的舌诊内容;下篇为建国后有关杂志舌诊论文的摘录。书末尚附有部分国外舌诊研究的论述,以及舌诊彩色图谱300余幅。本书内容广博,集古今舌诊文献之大全,对我国临床及舌诊研究都有重要参考价值,是一部具有较高实用价值的工具书和参考书。

(16) *Encyclopedia of China Tongue Inspection*, published by Academy Publishing House in February,1994, was compiled by Li Naimin. This book was divided into three parts, the first part was a ancient china medical book on tongue inspection which systematically arranged and researched tongue inspection from the dynasty prior to Qin, and West Han dynasty to 1949, the second part contents included tongue inspection and non-tongue inspection after the people's republic of china was founded, the third part was an abstract of relevant theses and magazines about tongue inspection after the people's republic of china was founded. At the end of book is an appendit of some abroad treatises about tongue inspection research, and more than 300 color photo on tongue inspection. This book contents are an extensive collection of ancient and modern medical documents on tongue inspection, and afforded a great reference value on our clinic and tongue inspection research, so this book was a highly practical reference book.

(17)《临床舌诊图谱与疾病治疗》翁维良主编,学苑出版社1997年1月出版,该书以历代有关舌诊著书为源流,综合现代舌诊研究工作,拍摄各种彩色病理舌彩图120幅,附有病例分析,并提出辨证施治及治疗处方。

(17) *Clinic Tongue Atlas And Treatment of Diseases*, published by Academy Publishing House in January,1997, was compiled by Weng Weiliang. This book contained monograph on tongue inspection in successive dynasties and synthesized modern researches on tongue inspection appended 120-color photo of pathogenic tongue and analysis of cases, the authors listed treatment based on syndrome differentiation and therapeutic formulas.

(18)《舌下络脉诊法的基础与临床研究》靳士英主编,广东科技出版社1998年3月出版,该书首先论述舌下络脉诊法源流、演变与传统理论,然后介绍了临床应用观察结果。照片及线条图200余幅,填补了此前舌诊图谱缺乏舌下络脉诊的空白。

(18) *The Foundation And Clinic Researches on Diagnosis of Vessels Below Tongue*, published by Guangdong Scientific Technology Publishing House in March, 1998, was compiled by Jin Shiying. This work firstly stated the origin, evolvement and traditional theory of vessels below tongue diagnosis, then introduced clinic application and result of observation., and appended 200 photos. So this work filled in the gaps in tongue atlas, which lacked vessels below tongue diagnosis.

(19)《舌诊源鉴》王季藜等主编,人民卫生出版社2001年9月出版,该书依据历代有关舌诊著书为源流,及历代医籍论述舌诊之精华,应用中西医结合理论,结合教学、临床与科研实践经验的总结,系统地介绍了舌象的发病机制,诊法及治疗方法,是一部中西医舌诊学专著。

(19) *Original Differentiation of Tongue Inspection*, published by the people's hygiene publishing house, was compiled by Wang jili. This book systematically introduced pathogenesis of tongue pictures, diagnostics and treatments on the basis of successive dynasties' medical books on tongue inspection and essences on tongue inspection of successive dynasties' medical books, integrating T.C.M and West Medicine, combining teaching and clinic and summary of scientific researches.

此外,还有一些古代医著虽非舌诊专书,但均有讨论舌诊的专篇章节,且颇有建树,堪称佳作。如李梴《医学入门》(1575年)的四诊部分、王肯堂《证治准绳》(1597年)舌诊部分、张介宾《景岳全书·舌色辨》(1624年)、陈士铎《石室秘录·伤寒辨舌秘法》(1687年)、林之翰《四诊抉微》(1723年)舌诊部分、张石顽《伤寒绪论·辨舌》(1795年)、吴坤安《伤寒指掌·察舌辨症歌》(1776年)、江笔花《笔花医镜·望舌色》(1824年)、章楠《医门棒喝·辨舌苔》(1825年)、汪宏《望诊遵经·望舌诊法提纲》(1875年)、周学海《周氏医学丛书·舌质舌苔辨》(1894年)等,有不少关于舌诊的精辟见解和宝贵经验。此外,温病学派在温病学说建立的过程中确立和丰富了"温病察舌"的经验,如吴有性的《温疫论》(1624年)、叶桂的《温热论》(1746年)、薛雪的《湿热论》(1754年)、余霖的《疫疹一得》(1794年)、陈平伯的《外感温病篇》(1824年)、吴瑭的《温病条辨》(1798年)、王孟英的《温热经纬》(1852年)等,都从各自的实践予以丰富、充实、完善了温病学说,并创立了一套适用于整个温热病的察舌方法,将舌诊和卫气营血辨证、三焦辨证联系在一起,从而奠定了温病察舌辨证施治的原则。

In addition, some medical works which were not monographs on tongue inspection also had chapters or sections discussing tongue inspection, and they all gave full play to theirs professional knowledge and are excellent works. For example, four diagnostics part of *ABC of Medicine* by LiYan(1575), tongue inspection part in *Standard of Syn-Drome And Treatment* by Wang Kentang(1597), *Jingyue's Complete Works·Differentiation of Tongue Color* by Zhang Jiebin(1624), *Secret Record in Stone Chamber·Secret Methods for Differentiating Tongue on Cold Attack* by ChenShiduo(1687), tongue inspection part in *The Concise Content of Diagnostic Methods* by LinZhihan(1723), *Introduction of Cold-Attack·Differentiating Tongue* by Zhang Shiwan(1795), *The Guide of The Treatise on Cold Attack·Song of Differentiating Syndrome by Inspecting Tongue* by Wu kunan(1776), *Bihua Medical Mirror·Inspecting Tongue Color* by Jiang Bihua, *Warning of Medicine·Differentiating Coating* by Zhang Nan(1825), *Observation Diagnosis by Adhering to Classics·Outline of Tongue Inspection* by Wang Hong(1875), *Zhou's Medical Series·Differentiating Tongue Texture And Tongue Coating* by Zhou xuehai(1894),etc, there are plenty of penetrating views and valuable experience. Besides, school of febrile diseases established and enriched experience of "inspecting tongue on febrile disease" in the course of its foundation, for example, *Treatise on Pestilence* by Wu Youxing(1624), *Treatise on Warm-Heat* by Ye Gui

(1746), *Treatise on Damp-Heat* by Xue Xue (1754), *A View of Pestilence with Rashes* by YuLing (1794), *Exogenous Febrile Diseases* by Chen Pingbo (1824), *Treatise on Differentiation And Treatment of Febrile Diseases* by Wu Tang (1798), *A Compendium on Febrile Diseases* by Wang Mengying, they all enriched, supplemented, and perfected febrile disease, and established a method of inspecting tongue applicable to whole febrile diseases, they combined the tongue inspection with Wei-qi-ying-xue syndrome and triple-jiao, therefore, they established a principle for treatment and syndrome differentiation by tongue inspection.

第一章 舌诊概要
Chapter one Abstract

临床实践证明,在疾病的发展过程中,舌象的变化迅速而又明显,它犹如窥视人体内脏生理功能与病理变化的一面镜子。凡脏腑的虚实、气血的盛衰、津液的盈亏、胃气的存亡、病情的浅深、病邪的性质、预后的吉凶,都能较为客观地从舌象上反映出来。由于舌诊在临床上有很大的诊断价值,舌诊已成为医生诊病的重要依据,是中医独具特色的诊法之一。

A long term clinical practice suggests the change of tongue has character of change and evidence in the course of disease. It is just like a mirror, which reflects physiological function and pathological changes of visceral. The excess and deficiency of the visceral, the exuberance or decline of *Qi* and blood, the wax or wane of body-fluid, the existence or exhaustion of *Stomach-Qi*, the deep or shallow location of disease, the mature of disease and the favorable or unfavorable condition of prognosis, all can be reflected objectively by tongue. Tongue inspection has a unique significance in clinic diagnosis of traditional Chinese medicine (TCM) and has become one of the important references for doctors to diagnose diseases.

第一节 舌诊原理
Section 1 The Mechanism of Tongue Inspection

1. 舌的形态结构和生理功能
1. Structures and Physiological Function of Tongue

(1) 形态结构
(1) Structures

舌是口腔中重要器官之一,它附着于口腔底部、下颌骨、舌骨,呈扁平而长形。舌为肌性器官,由黏膜和纵横交错的横纹肌组成,故《灵枢·经脉》说:"唇舌者,肌肉之本也"。

Tongue is one of important organs in the buccal cavity and attached by muscles to the lower jawbone and hyoid bone. It is flat and long, and belongs to a muscular organ that is formed by mucosa membrane and striated muscle. Thus, meridians, *The Chap-*

ter in Spirit Pirot Says,"The lips and tongue are the function of muscle."

舌的外形,舌的上面称舌背,下面称舌底。舌背又分为舌体与舌根两部分,以人字沟为分界(图1.1.1.1)。

The feature of tongue includes tongue back and tongue bottom. Tongue back is divided into two Part-tongue including body and tongue root, which are Bordered by *a Gulf in Middle Surface of Tongue*, shaped-like "人" (See color fig. 1.1.1.1).

舌体的前端(游离端)称为舌尖[1],舌体的后部人字形界沟之前称为舌根[2],舌体的中部称为舌中[3],舌体的两边称为舌边[4]。舌面的正中有一条不甚明显的纵行为纹,称为舌正中沟[5](图 1.1.1.2)。

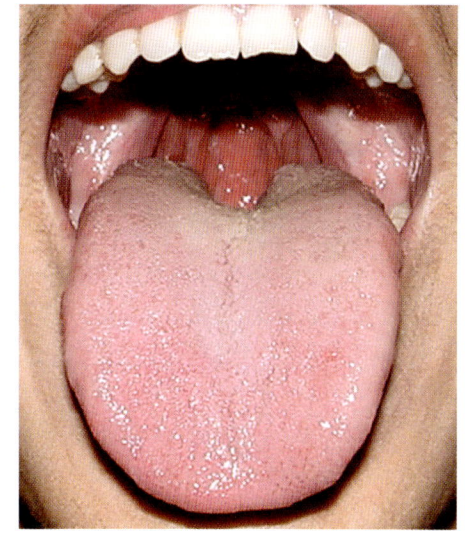

图(See color fig)1.1.1.1

Anterior tongue is called tongue tip[1] while the posterior is known as tongue root[2], The middle[3] of tongue is tongue-middle and the margins of tongue are described tongue-margin[4]. There is a vague striation in the middle of the surface of tongue, which is defined as Tongue-middle-gulf[5] (See color fig. 1.1.1.2).

当舌上卷时,可看到舌底。舌底正中线上有一条连于口腔底的皱襞,叫舌系带。舌系带左右两侧,有两根较粗大的舌下静脉,前人称之为舌下络脉(图1.1.1.3)。系带终点两侧各有一个小圆形突起,叫舌下肉阜,其顶部有舌下腺和颌下腺的共同开口,中医称其左侧的为金津,右侧的为玉液,是胃津、肾液上潮的孔道。

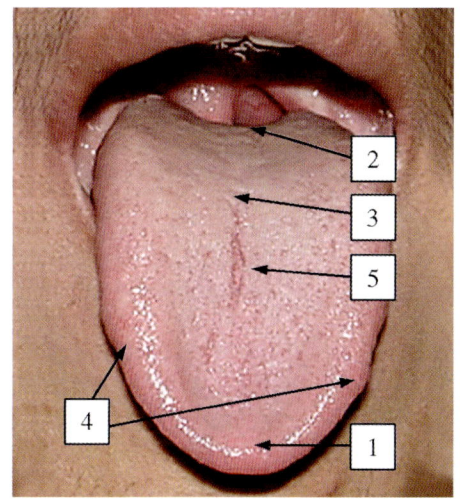

图(See color fig) 1.1.1.2

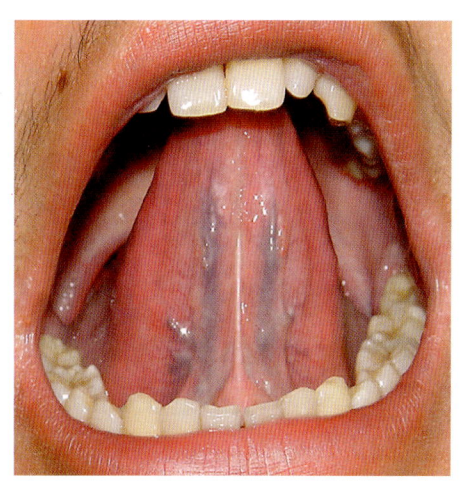

图(See color fig). 1.1.1.3

When tongue rises upward, its bottom is seen. A ruga, in the middle boundary of it, is attached to the bottom of buccal cavity, is called frenulum of tongue. There are two long hypoglossal vessels, on both on sides of the frenulum of the tongue. The sublingual caruncle is located at the end of the frenulum of tongue and its top is a common pore to the sublingual gland and submandibular Gland, the left is called Gold-Like fluid and the Right is Jade-like essence. The pore is the passageway that stomach fluid and kidney essence goes upward to the tongue (See color fig. 1.1.1.3).

舌面上覆盖着一层半透明的黏膜,舌背黏膜粗糙,形成许多突起,构成舌乳头。根据形状不同,舌乳头分为丝状乳头[1]、蕈状乳头[2]、轮廓乳头[3]和叶状乳头[4]四种。其中丝状乳头与蕈状乳头对舌象的形成有着密切的联系,轮廓乳头、叶状乳头与味觉有关(图1.1.1.4)。

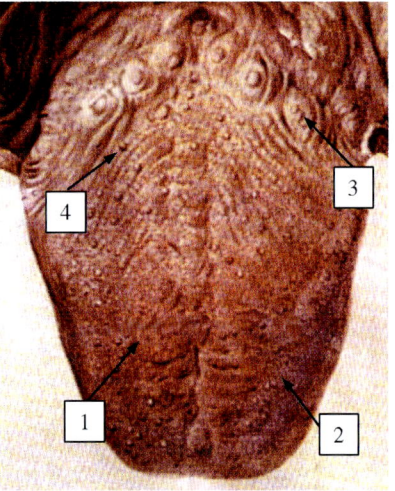

图(See color fig). 1.1.1.4

The tongue is covered with a semitransparent mucous membrane, which is very rough on its Back. A series of cone-shaped small projections called tongue papillae are located on the tongue back, also. There are four kinds papillae: filiform papillae[1], fungiform papillae[2], circumvallate papillae[3] and foliate papillae[4]. The front two play important role in forming tongue pictures, while the latter two have connection with taste (See color fig. 1.1.1.4).

丝状乳头数目最多,分布在舌尖、舌体和舌边,呈细长圆锥形,高2~3mm(图1.1.1.5)。它的复层扁平上皮常有角化和脱落,再混以食物残渣、唾液等,使舌黏膜表面覆以一层白色薄苔,称舌苔(图1.1.1.6)。此处上皮的形状和颜色,常随健康情况而发生改变。

The number of the filiform papillae is much more than others', distributing on the tongue tip, tongue body and tongue margins. Its shape is cylindrical and the height is about 2~3 mm(See color fig. 1.1.1.5). Those stratified squamous epithelium are often cornificated and deciduous, mixing with the retention of food and saliva, form a thin and white fur called tongue coating (See color fig. 1.1.1.6). The colors and shapes of epithelium will change as the condition of health does.

蕈状乳头数目较少,多见于舌尖,散在于丝状乳头之间,呈蕈状,基部窄而顶端钝圆。上皮表面比较平滑,有时可见有味蕾存在,固有膜中血管丰富,故乳头呈红色(图1.1.1.7);肉眼观察呈红色小点(图1.1.1.8)。蕈状乳头的形态及色泽改变,是舌质变化的主要因素。

The number of the fungiform papillae is small. It covers near to tongue tip and di-

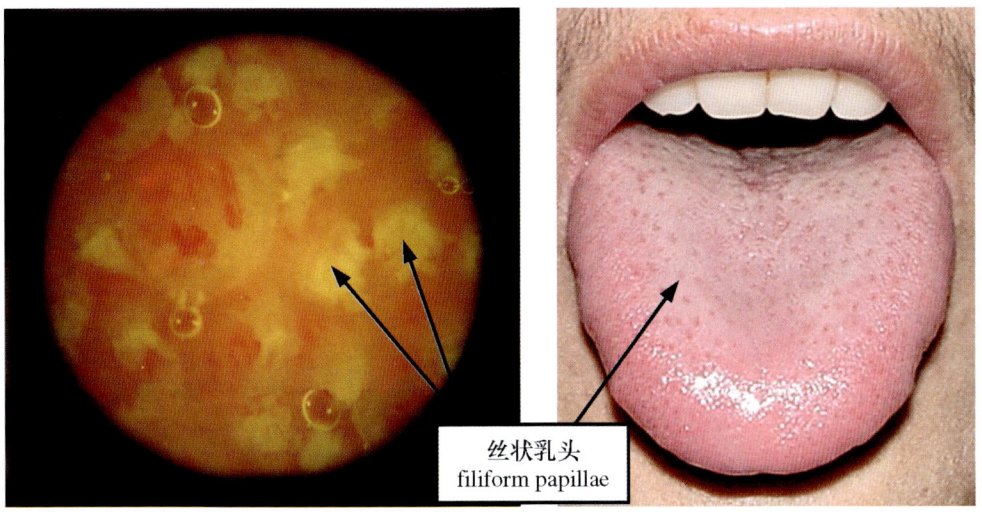

图(See color fig)1.1.1.5　　　　　图(See color fig)1.1.1.6

丝状乳头 filiform papillae

vides among the filiform papillae, shaped-like a fungus. Its basis is narrow, the top is circular, and the surface of epithelium is smooth. Sometimes, taste bud can be seen. Full of vessels in fixed main branch, this pupillae is red(See color fig. 1.1.1.7)., and look like red-point by gross examination (See color fig. 1.1.1.8). The change of texture and color is main factors of tongue texture.

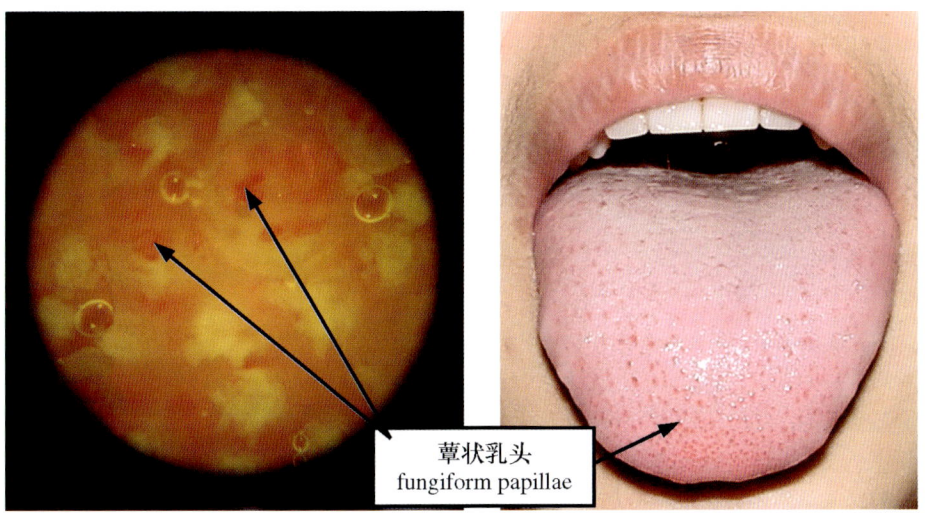

蕈状乳头 fungiform papillae

图(See color fig)1.1.1.7　　　　　图(See color fig)1.1.1.8

(2) 生理功能

(2) Function

舌具有搅拌食物,感受味觉和调节语音的功能。

Tongue has function of mastication, feeling taste and regulating voice.

舌作为一个肌性器官,能自主灵活的伸缩卷转,使食物在口腔内得到充分的搅拌。

舌的轮廓乳头和叶状乳头内含味觉神经末梢,能充分感受味觉。《中藏经·论小肠虚实寒热生死逆顺脉证之法》说:"舌之官也,和则能言而机关利健,善别其味也"。《彩图辨舌指南·舌之乳头》特别指出:"在舌根近旁,排列如人字形,较前数种为大,内藏味觉神经之末梢,曰味蕾"。舌的灵活自主运动,能配合胸腔、声带的发音,使语音清晰流畅。

As a muscular organ, The tongue can moves smartly, as a result, food can be masticated throughout in the buccal cavity. In addition, there are lots of nerve endings in the outer circumvallate papilla and foliate papillae, which help the tongue to feel taste completely. *Methods for Diagnosing the Deficiency and Excess, Cold and Heat, Existence and Exhaustion of Small Intestine, in Zhong Zang Classic* says, "If the tongue is functioning harmoniously, it is coherent to speech and good to distinguish the flavor." Lingual papilla, *The Chapter of Guides for Tongue Diagnosis* states, "Taste bud is near the tongue root, shaped like '人', larger than others', and full of taste nerve endings. The movement, the pronounce of the thorax and vocal cords, make speech clear and fluent."

2. 舌与脏腑经络、气血津液的关系
2. The Relationship Between Tongue and Viscera, Meridians *Qi-Blood*, and Body Fluid

舌虽是口腔内的一个局部器官,但与脏腑经络、气血津液有着密切的联系。

The tongue is a local organ in the buccal cavity, it is closely related to viscera, meridians, *qi*, *blood* and body fluid.

(1) 舌与脏腑经络的关系
(1) Tongue, Viscera and Meridians

舌体通过经络与许多的内在脏器相联系,舌为心之苗,《灵枢·脉度》说:"心气通于舌,心和则舌能知五味矣"。《灵枢·经脉》曰:"手少阴之别,……循经入于心,系舌本";因心主血脉,而舌的脉络丰富,心血上荣于舌,故人体气血运行情况,可反映在舌质的颜色上;心主神明,舌体的运动又受心神的支配,因而舌体运动是否灵活自如,语言是否清晰,与神志密切相关。故舌与心、神的关系极为密切,可以反映心、神的病变(图 1.1.2.1)。

The tongue connects visceral with the help of many meridians. It's the sprout of the heart. The *heart-qi* corresponds with the tongue, if it's functio-

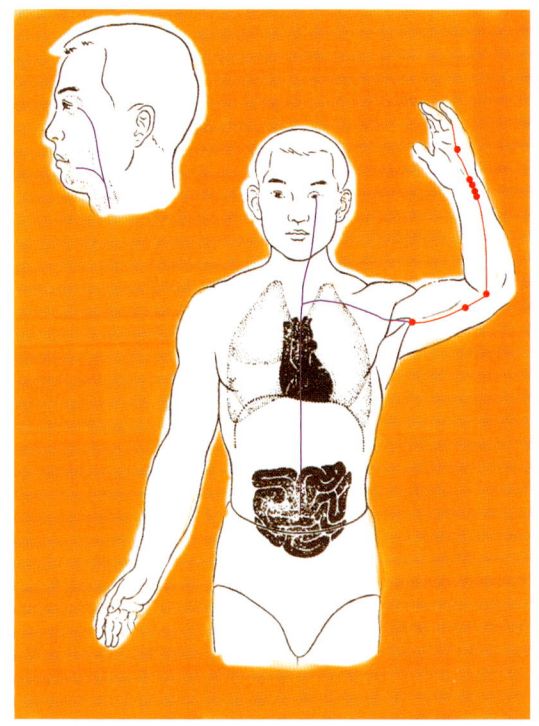

图(See color fig)1.1.2.1

ning harmoniously, the tongue can feel five kinds of flavors. *Meridians*, one of *The Chapter in Sprint Pirot* says, "*Shao-Yin Meridians of Hand*, passes through the heart and links the tongue." The heart dominates the blood and vessels, which are abundant under the tongue; heart-blood rises upward to nourish the tongue. So circulation of the *qi* and blood can be reflected by tongue texture. As the heart dominates the mind, and the mind commands tongue, the tongue has closely connected with the mind. Therefore, the tongue, the heart and the mind all can be reflected by tongue picture (See color fig. 1.1.2.1).

舌为脾之外候。足太阴脾经连舌本、散舌下,舌居口中司味觉,而《灵枢·脉度》说:"脾气通于口,脾和则口能知五谷矣。"故曰脾开窍于口。《灵枢·经脉》曰:"脾足太阴之脉,……连舌本,散舌下";中医学认为,脾主运化、化生气血。舌体赖气血充养,舌象能反映气血的盛衰,而与脾主运化、化生气血的功能直接相关(图1.1.2.2)。

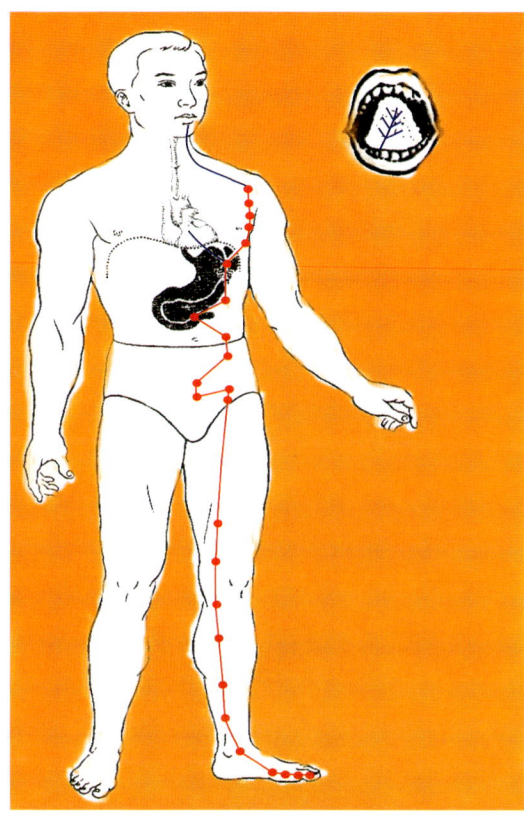

图(See color fig)1.1.2.2

The tongue is regarded as the out show of the spleen. *Tai-Yin Meridians of Foot* links the tongue that dominates taste. Those points can be supported by some quotations. For example, *Meridians, the Chapter of Sprint Pirot* points out, "*Tai-Yin Meridians* link the tongue." (Another saying) in *Meridians, the Chapter of Sprint Pirot* states, "*Spleen-qi* passes through the mouth, if the spleen is functioning harmoniously then the mouth can feel the five kinds of flavors." In TCM, the spleen dominates transportation and transformation, the normal tongue depends heavily upon the nourishment of *qi* and blood, so, the tongue reflects the exuberance and decline of *qi* and blood, and relates to the spleen (See color fig. 1.1.2.2).

肝藏血、主筋,肾藏精。《灵枢·经脉》曰:"肝者,筋之合也,筋者,聚于阴器,而脉络于舌本也","肾足少阴之脉,……其直者,从肾上贯肝膈,入肺中,循喉咙,夹舌本"(图1.1.2.3);足太阳膀胱经经筋结于舌本;肺系上达咽喉,与舌根相连。肺、肠、胆虽无本经经脉直接通于舌,但通过经脉手足同经的影响,也与舌有间接联系。另外,舌居于口腔之中,与食道相连,故与胃也有着直接连属关系。因而脏腑一旦发生病变,舌象也会出现相应的变化。所以观察舌象的变化,可以测知内在脏腑的病变。

The liver stores blood and dominates the tendons, while the kidney stores essence. Thus, *Meridians*, one of *Chapter in Sprint Pirot* says, "The liver corresponds with the tendons, which assemble on urethra and genitals, and its meridians links the tongue." "*Shao-Yin Meridians of Foot*, goes upward and rounds the diaphragm, passes through the long, cross the throat and links the tongue." *The Lung Meridians* passes through pharynx and connects with the tongue. The lung, the intestine, and the gallbladder, have associated with the tongue indirectly. With the help of attached meridians. In addition, the tongue joints the esophagus, and connects the stomach with the aid of the esophagus. Therefore, the disease of viscera can be diagnosed by tongue-observation (See color fig. 1.1.2.3).

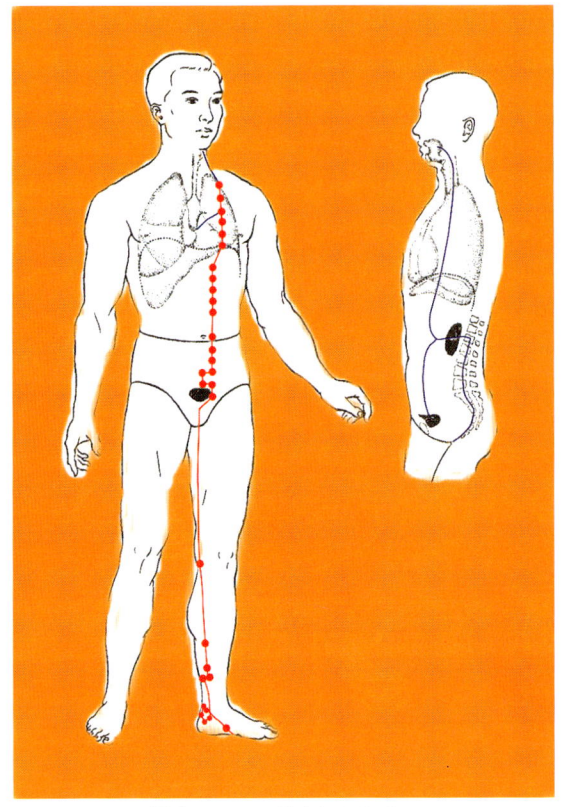

图(See color fig)1.1.2.3

(2) 舌与气血津液的关系
(2) The connectio of tongue with, *Qi*, Blood and Body Fluid

心主血为五脏六腑之大主,脾藏营而为诸脏后天之本。舌为心之苗窍、脾之外候,故诸脏营血之盈亏必显于舌(图1.1.2.4)、(图1.1.2.5)。舌上之苔,为胃气熏蒸水谷浊气上潮所生,诸腑气化之动静亦易显于苔(图1.1.2.6)、(图1.1.2.7)。另外,舌下有金津、玉液,为胃津肾液上潮之孔道,如《灵枢·胀论》所曰:"廉泉玉英者,津液之道也"。故津液之多少,亦显现于舌(图1.1.2.8)(图1.1.2.9)。

The heart dominates the blood and it's the supreme monarch of all organs. The spleen stores the nutritive blood, and it is the foundation of acquired constitution. The tongue is the sprout of the heart and out-shows of the spleen. So the wax and wane of blood can be manifested by tongue (See color fig. 1.1.2.4) (See color fig. 1.1.2.5). Tongue coating, produced by steaming stomach *qi*, exhibits function of the viscera (See color fig. 1.1.2.6) (See color fig. 1.1.2.7). In addition, under the tongue is common pore, by which the stomach fluid and kidney essence flow upwards. It is called *Gold-like fluid* and *Jade-like fluid* in TCM. Just like *Theory of Distension*, *the Chapter in Spirit Pirot* says, "The *Gold-like fluid* and *Jade-like fluid* is the passageway for the stomach fluid and kidney essence. The flourish and withering of the body fluid can be reflected on the tongue." (See color fig. 1.1.2.8) (See color fig. 1.1.2.9).

第一章 舌诊概要

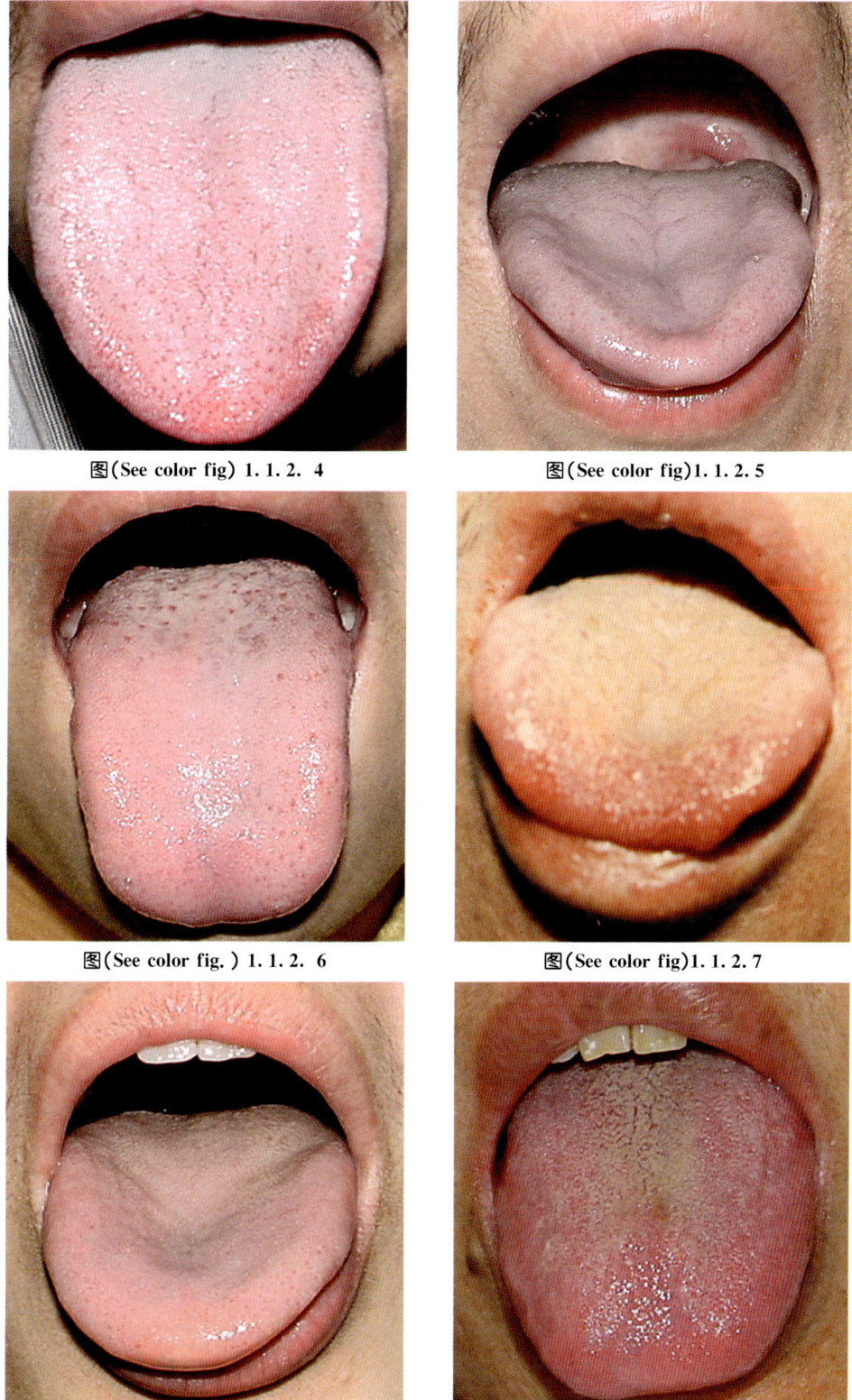

图(See color fig) 1.1.2.4　　　　　　　图(See color fig) 1.1.2.5

图(See color fig.) 1.1.2.6　　　　　　　图(See color fig) 1.1.2.7

图(See color fig) 1.1.2.8　　　　　　　图(See color fig) 1.1.2.9

脏腑的病变反映于舌面,舌诊候病的基本规律,古代医籍有不同的划分记载,其中比较一致的说法是:舌质候五脏病变为主,侧重血分;舌苔候六腑病变为主,侧重气分。舌尖多反映上焦心肺的病变;舌中多反映中焦脾胃的病变;舌根多反映下焦肾的病变;舌两侧多反映肝胆的病变。

　　There are many records about the basic laws of tongue-observation, and that "the change of tongue reflects inner visceral change". The ancient statements on this were different. The most popular was, "The tongue texture reflects mainly disease of *the Five Zang-Viscera* while the tongue coating reflects mainly *the Six-Fu Viscera*. The tongue tip belongs to the heart, the middle to spleen and stomach; the root to the kidney and the bilateral margins to the liver and gallbladder."

　　总之,舌体虽小,但由于它与脏腑经络气血津液的紧密联系,故能客观、灵敏地反映它们的生理功能和病理变化。正如《伤寒指掌·察舌辨症法》所说:"病之经络、脏腑、营卫、气血、表里、阴阳、寒热、虚实,毕形于舌"。《临证验舌法》曰:"舌者心之苗也,五脏六腑之大主,其气通于此,其窍开于此也,查诸脏腑图,脾、肺、肝、肾无不系根于心,核诸经络,考手足阳明,无脉不通于舌。则知经络脏腑之病,不独伤寒发热有苔可验,即凡内伤杂证,也无一不呈其形、着其色于舌"。

　　In conclusion, the tongue is small, and it is closely related to viscera and meridians, *qi* and blood, and fluid. So it can reflect physiological function and pathological change objectively and smartly. *Tongue Diagnosis the Chapter in Prescription on Cold-Attack*, points out, "All diseases can be exhibited on the tongue, whatever the disease exists in meridians and viscera, *Yin* and *Wei-stage*, *qi* and blood, and whatever it belongs to exogenous and interior (syndrome, *yin* and *yang*, cold and heat, deficiency and excess." *Tongue Diagnosis for Clinical Practice* also states, "The tongue is the sprout of the heart, the message of *the Five Zang-Viscera* and *Six-Fu Viscera*. The *heart-qi* crosses the tongue and often into the tongue. Thus, the ailment of the viscera and meridians communicate with the tongue."

第二节　舌诊的方法与注意事项
Section 2　Method and Special attention on Observing Tongue

　　望舌是对舌的整体形象进行系统观察,舌象变化虽多,但若能掌握操作的基本方法和舌象特征的一般意义,就能达到执简驭繁、知常达变之目的。

　　Tongue observation is observing the whole tongue picture systematically. Although the tongue picture is varied, the doctor can analyze pathogenesis, summarize syndrome, and understand abnormal changes, if he masters the basic method and the characteristics of tongue.

1. 舌诊的基本操作
1. The Method of Tongue-Examination

舌诊是以望舌为主,有时还须辅助舌觉之问诊和扪摸揩刮之切诊等进行。

Tongue-examination mainly refers to tongue observation. Sometimes interrogation and palpation, which includes touching, feeling, scrubbing and scraping, is also necessary for clinic diagnosis.

(1) 望舌的基本姿势
(1) Posture

望舌时,要求患者面朝自然光线,一般采取正坐位(重病患者可以仰卧),头略扬起,尽量张开口,使光线直照口中,再让患者将舌伸出口外,并使舌体自然舒张,舌面展开呈扁平形,舌尖略向下弯,便于观察(图1.2.1.1)。医者站立或对面正坐,姿势可略高于患者,以便俯视患者口舌部位(图1.2.1.2)。

When observing tongue, the patient should face the natural light and sit up right (patient with serious disease can lie on his back), with head lifted slightly, and mouth open enough, so as the natural light reaches the buccal cavity and the tongue can be inspected carefully. Doctor also should ask patient to stretch out tongue, relax the tongue, and flatten the tough with tongue tip winding down. All these are favorable to observe carefully (See color fig. 1.2.1.1). On the other hand, doctor ought to stand or sit in the position right opposite to the patient (See color fig. 1.2.1.2).

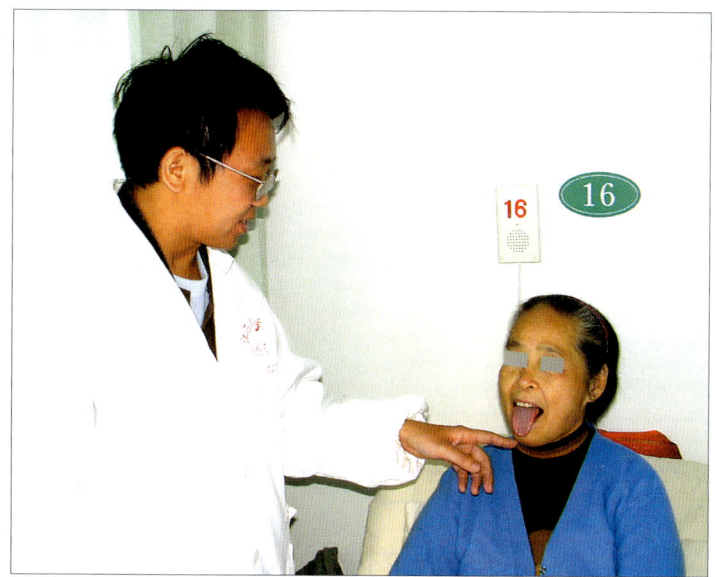

图(See color fig)1.2.1.1

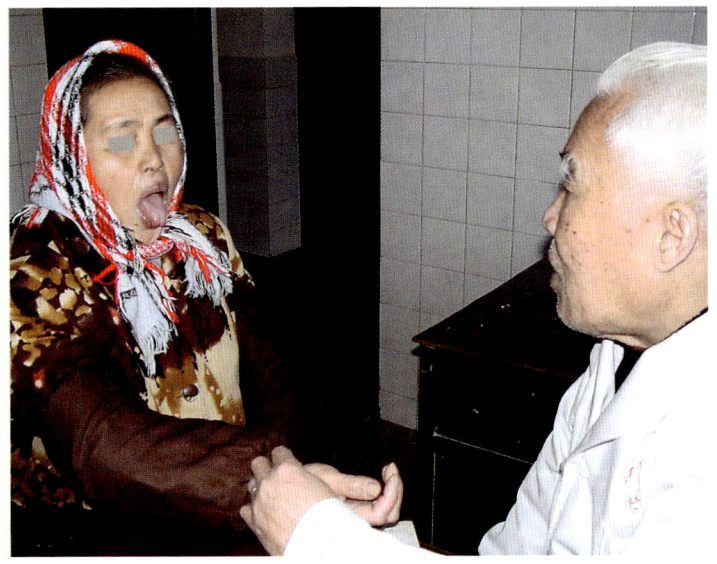

图(See color fig)1.2.1.2

伸舌时,要求病人使舌体自然放松,忌用拙力,以免舌体紧张、卷曲而变形,致使舌色加深发暗、舌苔紧凑变样(图1.2.1.3)。同时,伸舌时间不宜过久,以免影响舌体血液循环而使舌质渐转青紫。《辨舌指南·辨舌之苔垢》就曾指出:平人舌质淡红,偶因用力过度,会骤变深红。无病之舌,由于伸舌姿势不同,或紧或尖,或松或软,或收束紧而成尖锋(图1.2.1.4)。对于这类患者,可反复训练几次,使之学会放松舌体,充分展平。

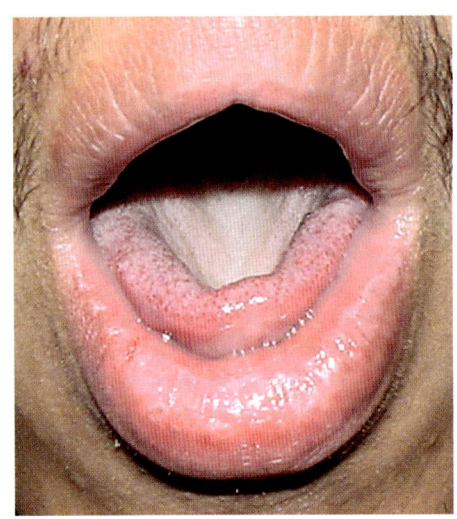

图(See color fig)1.2.1.3

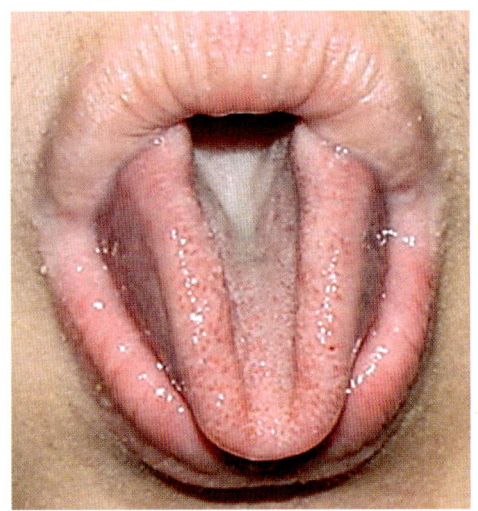

图(See color fig)1.2.1.4

As to stretching tongue, special attention should be paid to some points. When stretching out the tongue, the patient should make sure the tongue is relaxed, to avoid the over extension and curve of the tongue, so as not make effect on the color becoming darker, and the coating constricting (See color fig. 1.2.1.3). At the same time, the time used for stretching shouldn't be too long, because it affects blood circulation of the tongue, which makes tongue texture turn to bluish purple. Tongue coating, the chapter in *Guides for Tongue Diagnosis* says, Pink is the normal color, however, it is easy to change into crimson with much strength. As the posture of stretching tongue is different, tongue coating can show different features, such as tightness, sharpness, looseness and softness, even spire caused by contribution excessively (See color fig. 1.2.1.4). Those patients can be trained several times to learn to relax and flatten tongue body completely.

(2) 望舌的基本顺序
(2) The Basic Procedure of Tongue-Observing

望舌的顺序是先看舌尖,再看舌中、舌边,最后看舌根,依次扫视;先察舌体,再察舌苔,以免伸舌较久舌体色泽失真。再就根据舌体、舌苔的各自基本特征,分项考察。

The procedure is tongue tip is first, then the middle, the bilateral margins, and last is the root. When observing tongue texture, tongue body is first, followed by tongue coating, so as not to make them false, if the time for stretching is too tonged. According the individual characters of tongue body and coating, doctor diagnoses them step-by-step.

察舌体,主要从舌质的颜色、光泽、形状和动态几方面着眼;察舌苔,主要从舌苔的有无、色泽、质地和分布状态几方面考察。最后,有必要时,还须查看舌下静脉。

When doctor exams tongue texture, he should put emphasis on inspecting the abnormal changes of color, shape, and movement of tongue. Likewise, the color, quality and division are also main aspects for observing tongue coating. Sometimes, the veins under the tongue ought to be observed, if it needs to.

(3) 舌诊的辅助手法
(3) Aiding Method of Tongue-observing

① 扣舌、摸舌
① Toughing and Feeling

望舌有疑惑时,须配合其他诊察方法。如为了核实舌之润燥,须用扣舌摸舌以测之;扣舌摸舌时,医者应先洗净手,再用食指指腹轻触患者舌面(图1.2.1.5);扣舌须在舌面的一定部位点按2～3下,看指腹湿染的程度。

If suspecting symptoms during tongue observing, the doctor needs to combine other diagnosis methods. For example, touching and feeling are usually used to verity moistness and dryness of the coating. Before the procedure, the doctor should make sure his hands are clean, then, he can touch and feel the patient's tongue with the index finger (See color fig. 1.2.1.5). Palpating refers to pressing a certain position on the surface of tongue for 2～3 times.

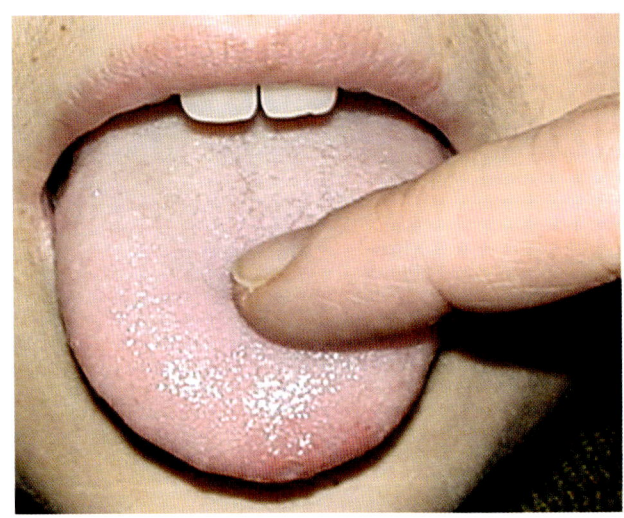

图(See color fig)1.2.1.5

摸舌则由舌根向舌尖方向滑动1～3次,不仅要视察指腹的湿染情况,有时还须体察舌面对指腹的刮刺感觉,以鉴别舌质舌苔的糙粘程度(图1.2.1.6)。

Touching refers to sliding your index finger from the root to the tip of tongue for 1~3 times. Touching and feeling are to distinguish moistness, dryness, and roughness and solidness of the tongue texture and coating (See color fig. 1.2.1.6).

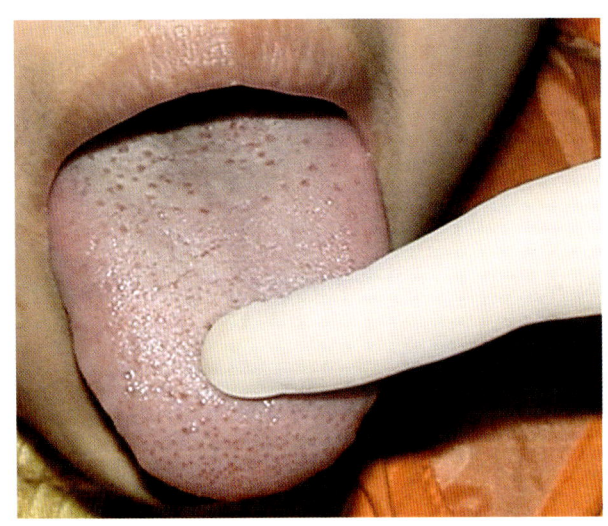

图(See color fig)1.2.1.6

② 揩舌、刮舌
② Scrubbing and Scraping

为了辨明苔之松紧、腐腻以及有无根底,须用揩舌刮舌以验之。舌望之干而扪之湿,为假燥现象,是湿阻气化而津失敷布之征;苔望之厚,揩之易退,为苔质松腐,而刮之不脱,为苔质紧腻;揩刮之后,苔底全无者为无根,苔减而不尽者为有根。《辨舌指南·辨舌之苔垢》指出:"苔之燥润糙粘,须以指摸为准"。

In clinic practice, scrubbing and scraping are mainly used to ascertain looseness, tense, putridness and greasiness, to diagnosis whether the tongue coating is root or non-rooted. It may look like dryness but moistness indeed when it is scraped. This kind of coating is called false coating. It is common of dampness obstructing *qi* and body fluid failing to metabolism. The coating called putrid coating looks thick and it is easy to exfoliate after being scraped. If the coating doesn't exfoliate, it is shown the coating is tight and greasy. If there is no coating on the tongue, it is called non-rooted. While only a little coating is still regarded as rooted coating. Tongue coating, *the Chapter in Guides for Tongue Diagnosis* points out, "The criterion for distinguish moistness, dryness, roughness and greasiness, should be decided by scrubbing and scraping."

刮舌时,须用经过消毒的刮舌板或压舌板,以适中的力量,由舌根向舌尖缓慢推刮,可连续3～5次(图1.2.1.7)。

When scraping the doctor ought to use a clear and sterilized sheet to scrape the coating slowly from the root to the tip of tongue. With moderate strength, it is allowed to do for 3～5 times (See color fig. 1.2.1.7).

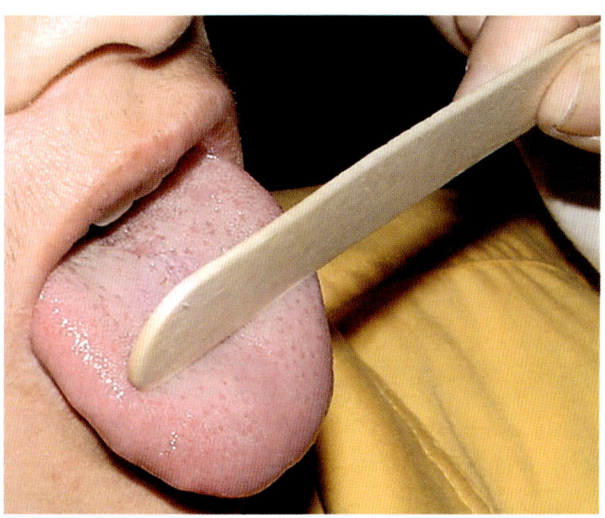

图(See color fig)1.2.1.7

揩舌时,须用消毒纱布一小块,卷于食指端,蘸少许清水或薄荷煎的水,以湿润为度,再从舌根向舌尖,连续揩拭4～5次(图1.2.1.8)。

In order to scrub correctly, a piece of disinfectant cloth is needed. The method is to use the cloth to wind around the index finger, soaked in clear water or peppermint water and scrub the tongue from the root to the tip. You had better to do that for 4～5times continually(See color fig. 1.2.1.8).

操作之中,刮舌、揩舌都须用力适当,过轻则应退之苔垢没能退去,过重则难退之苔垢亦强行退去,且易损伤舌体。刮揩之后,注意观察舌面苔垢的脱落、复生等情况。二者

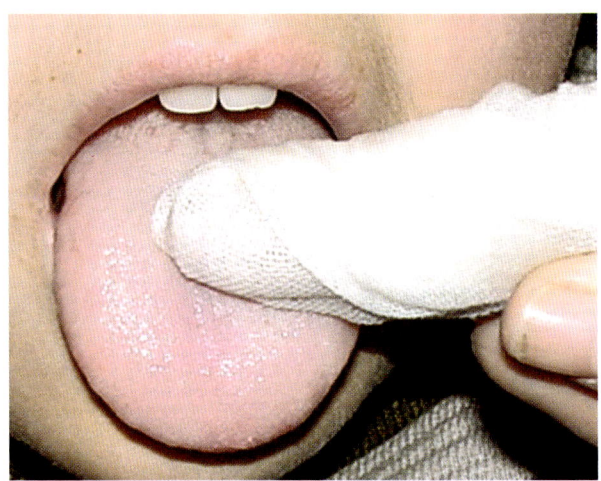

图 (See color fig)1.2.1.8

的诊断意义虽然相似,但刮舌着力较深,揩舌着力较浅,故前者较适用于紧敛厚腻之苔,后者较适用于浮露松腐之苔。一般多先用揩法,不效则再用刮法。

During procedure, the strength should be moderate, too little strength leads to the coating expected to scrape off still exist, while too much strength leads to the coating expected to keep exfoliate, besides, it is easy to injure the tongue. After scraping and scrubbing, the exfoliation and regeneration of coating are supposed to inspect carefully. Although the significance for diagnosis is similar, their requirements are different. Scraping requires much strength while scrubbing just a little. So scraping is suited to diagnose light coating, thick coating and greasy coating, and scrubbing suited for loose coating and putrid coating. Generally speaking, scrubbing is first, followed by scraping is it needs to.

另外,当舌苔疑有染色、粘物等假象时,应当结合问诊,询问有无饮食、服药及味觉异常等情况,予以鉴别处理。观察舌体动态时,可要求病人转舌、说话等,以便了解舌体是否灵活、有无歪斜等情况,并询问有无疼痛、麻木等感觉。

In addition, if food or drugs have dyed the coating colors, doctor should combine interrogation to get some information, such as diet, drugs and taste, etc. When observing movement of tongue, doctor may ask patient to turn around the tongue to speak, it is favorable to diagnose. Sometimes, interrogation, including pain, apoplexy and paraplegia should not be neglected, too.

2. 舌诊的注意事项
2. Special Attentions on observing Tongue

舌诊是中医临床诊病的重要依据,为保证其操作的正确性,所获信息的准确性,察舌时注意以下几点:

Tongue-examination is important basis of the clinic diagnosis. In order to secure the correct method and true message, special attentions should be paid to some points, which can make false changes in tongue picture.

(1) 光线条件

(1) Light

察舌首先要注意光线。因为光线对舌色的影响极大。同一舌象在不同的照明条件下会有效显著的色觉差异,稍有疏忽即易致错觉,导致误诊。正如《辨舌指南·观舌之心法》所云:"灯下看黄苔,每成白色,然则舌虽可凭,而亦未尽可凭,非细心审察,亦难免于误治矣。"

Light has serious effect on the color of tongue. It is the same color that can be looked as different color. Under the different light, of course, that often leads to mistakes. Just as *Prescription of Tongue-Observing*, *the Chapter in Guides for Tongue Diagnosis* says, "In lamp light, the yellow coating can be seen as a white coating, the tongue picture is important to diagnose, but it is not enough, doctor ought to inspect it carefully to avoid making mistakes."

光线条件,以昼日充足而柔和的自然光线为佳,让舌面正对光亮处(图1.2.2.1);要避免在暴日直射、阴天背光及有色灯光下察舌。

It is best to observe tongue in daytime under the full and soft natural light, because it is benefit for tongue examination (See color fig. 1.2.2.1). What is more, tongue observing should be away from strong light in the sun, week light in cloudy and lamp light with color.

(2) 食物或药品影响

(2) Diet and Drugs

饮食、药物等由口而入时,会对舌象产生直接的影响。

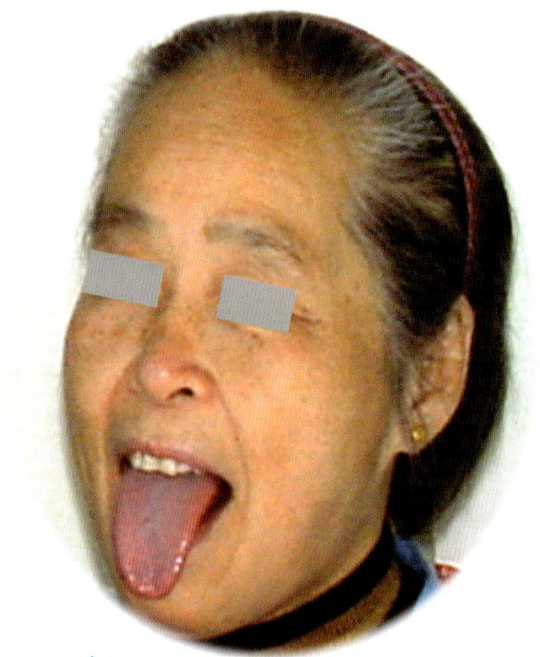

图(See color fig)1.2.2.1

Food and drugs can also influence tongue picture directly.

某些饮食、药物的着色物有染苔现象,如牛乳、豆浆等,可使舌苔发白变厚(图1.2.2.2);橘子、核黄素及中药汤剂,会使舌苔黄染(图1.2.2.3);酸梅汤、咖啡、含铁补品,以及长期吸烟等,会使舌苔呈褐色(图1.2.2.4)。

For example, milk and bean-mild can change coating into thick and white (See color fig. 1.2.2.2), orange, Vitamin B$_2$ and herb decoction, dye coating into yellow (See color fig. 1.2.2.3), and sweet-sour plum juice, coffee, nourishment filled with Fe^{2+}, and long-term smoking, all will turn coating color into black (See color fig1.2.2.4).

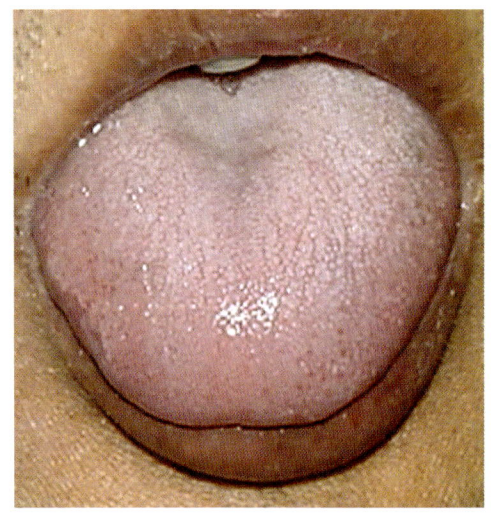

图(See color fig)1.2.2.2

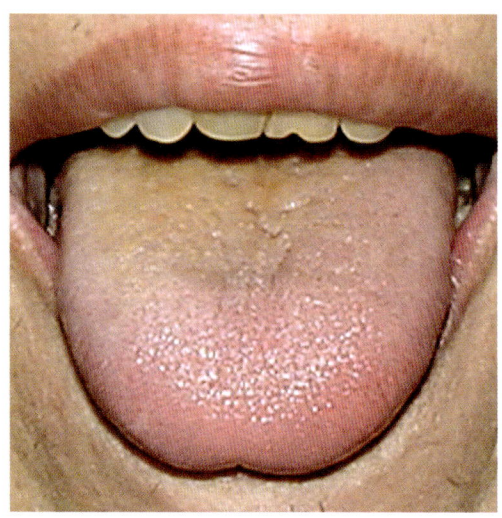

图(See color fig)1.2.2.3

某些刺激食物作用,如刚进辣椒、生姜等辛辣之品或过热、煎炸食物,会使舌质充血而红色加深(图1.2.2.5);长期服用某些抗生素,可导致黑腻苔或霉腐苔(图1.2.2.6)。

Some peppery and pungent food, like hot pepper, ginger and fried food, will redden the tongue body (See color fig. 1.2.2.5). Some antibiotics can also cause black and greasy coating or mould putrid coating (See color fig. 1.2.2.6).

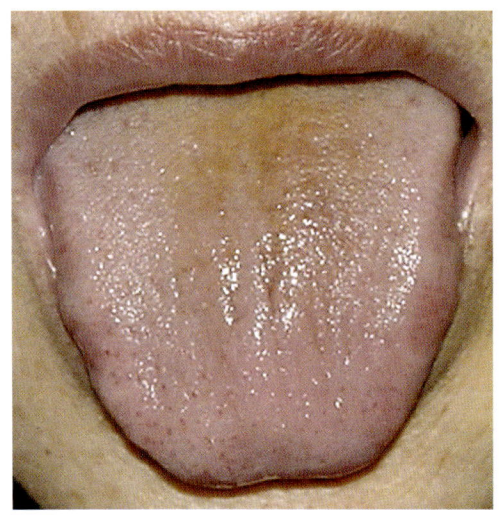

图(See color fig)1.2.2.4

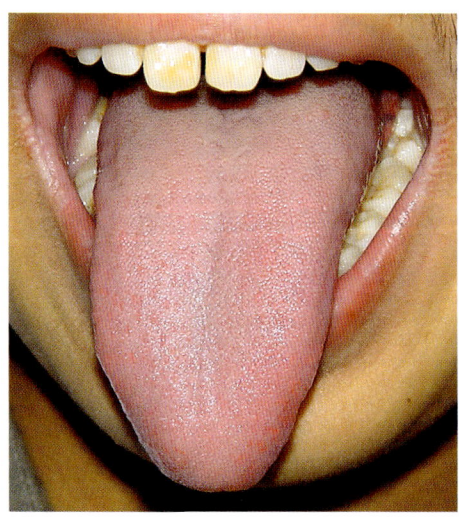

图(See color fig) 1.2.2.5

（3）口腔对舌象的影响
(3) Effect of Buccal Cavity

牙齿残缺,可造成同则舌苔偏厚(图 1.2.2.7);镶牙可使舌边留有齿痕(图 1.2.2.8)。

Loss of teeth can cause the coating becoming thicker at the same side (See color fig. 1.2.2.7), while inlaying teeth can produce teeth print on the bilateral margins of tongue (See color fig. 1.2.2.8).

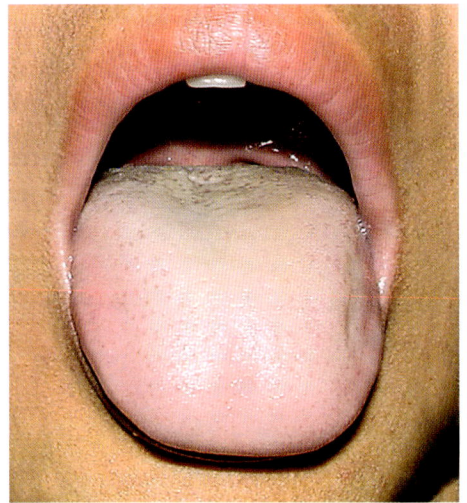

图(See color fig)1.2.2.6

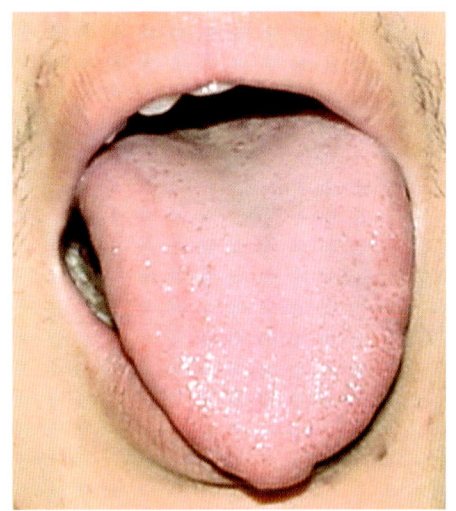

图(See color fig)1.2.2.7

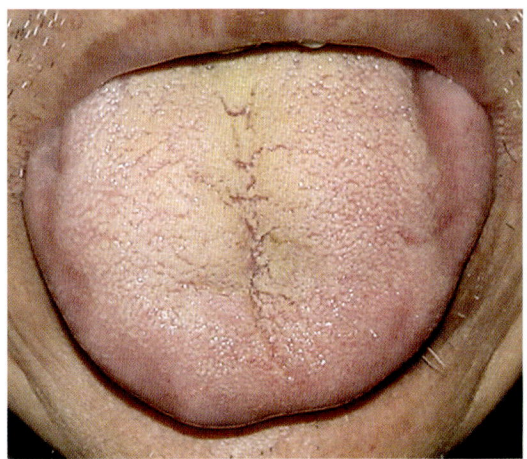

图(See color fig)1.2.2.8

第三节 舌诊的基本内容和正常舌象
Section 3　Content of Tongue Inspection and Normal Tongue

1. 舌诊的基本内容
1. Contents of Tongue Inspection

舌诊主要观察舌质与舌苔两个方面的变化。舌质又称舌体,是舌的肌肉和脉络等组织。诊察舌质主要观察舌神、舌色、舌形和舌态等方面的变化,以候脏腑之虚实,气血之盛衰。

Tongue Inspection includes observing tongue body (texture) and observing tongue coating. Tongue texture is the main body of the tongue and is made up of muscles and vessels (See color fig. 1.3.1.1). Observing tongue texture is observing the abnormal changes of the vitality, color, shape and movement of tongue body.

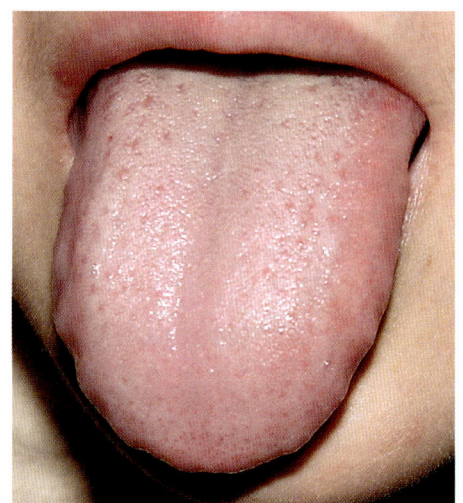

图(See color fig)1.3.1.1

舌苔是舌体上面附着的一层苔状物(图1.3.1.1),诊察舌苔主要观察苔色和苔质等方面的改变,以测病邪的性质、病位的浅深、邪正的消长。《辨舌指南》说:"辨舌质,可决五脏之虚实,视舌苔,可察六淫之浅深"。又说:"观舌质可验其证之阴阳虚实,审苔垢可知其邪之寒热浅深"。舌质与舌苔的综合变化,称为舌象。临床舌诊,只有综合分析舌象变化,才能全面了解病情,为诊断提供依据。

Tongue coating is thin fur-like on the tongue body in normal people (See color fig. 1.3.1.1). Observing tongue coating includes observing the color and the texture, so we know the nature of disease, the deep and shallow location of disease, the wax and wane of evil *qi* and *genuine-qi*, *Guides for Tongue Diagnosis* states, "The excess and deficiency of viscera, can be diagnosed through tongue texture, while the shallow and deep location of the six climatic evils through the coating", and saying, "The *yin* and *yang* excess and deficiency can be verified by observing texture, while the cold, heat, shallow and deep location of evils by observing coating." Those systemic change of tongue texture and coating is called tongue picture. It is through summarizing and analyzing the changes that we can understand disease completely, and supply correct information for clinic practice.

舌神有荣活与枯晦;舌色有淡红、淡白、红、绛、紫、青;舌形有胖瘦、老嫩、裂痕、点刺;

舌态有软硬、伸缩、歪斜、颤动等。

The tongue vitality is shown in the flourishing or withering of tongue texture, the tongue color includes pink, pale red, crimson, purple and blue, the tongue shape includes tenderness, toughness, corpulence swelling, thinness, crack and prickle, the movement statement includes stiffness, protruding and licking, wryness and tremor, etc.

舌苔《伤寒论》称之为"舌胎",《形色外诊简摩·伤寒舌苔辨证》则引《伤寒绪论》之言:"舌胎之名,始于长沙,以其邪气结,如有所怀,故谓之胎"。苔色有白、黄、灰、黑;苔质有厚薄、润燥、松紧 偏全、聚散、剥落、有根与无根等。

The tongue coating is called tongue embryo in *Treaties on Cold-Attack*. There is a paragraph quoted from *Introduction of Treaties Cold-Attack in Tongue Diagnosis on Cold-Attack*, *the Chapter of Summaries for Feature of Tongue* saying, "The tongue embryo is named by *Zhang ZhongJing* first, because *evil-qi* stagnates on the tongue and it's just like embryo. The color of coating includes white, yellow, greasy and black. The texture includes thickness, thinness, moistness, dryness, putrid and greasiness, even and uneven, exfoliation, wax and wane, root and non-root.

另外,在特殊情况下,还要参看舌下络脉,观察其长短、粗细、形状和颜色。

In addition, under the special condition, hypoglossal vessels including its length, diameter, shape and color, should be inspected carefully.

2. 正常舌象
2. The Normal Tongue Picture

要识别病态舌象,首先应掌握正常的舌象,知常才能达变。

In order to distinguish the abnormal changes of tongue, normal picture ought to be understood first.

正常舌象的特点是:舌体柔软灵活,舌色淡红明润,舌形大小适中,舌苔薄白均匀,苔质干湿适中,分布均匀有根而边尖略少。简称为"淡红舌,薄白苔"(图1.3.2.1)。

The normal tongue is characterized as a middle size, soft, neither tough nor tender, free moving, pink color, covered by thin and even white coating with moderate moistness, which

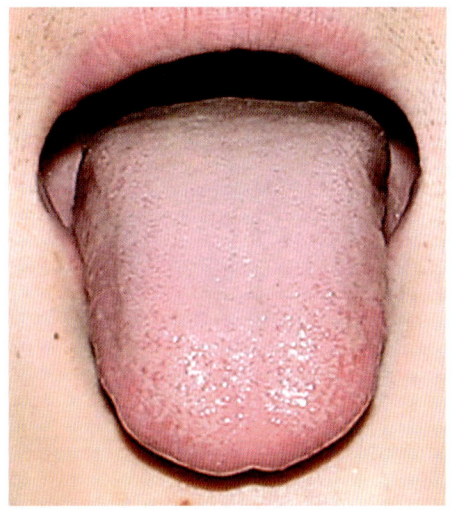

图(See color fig)1.3.2.1

could not be scraped away and has its root in tongue. It usually is summarized "Pink tongue with white and thin coating"(See color fig. 1.3.2.1).

正常舌象形成的原理,《舌胎统志》认为:"舌为心之苗,其色当红,红不娇艳,其质当泽,泽非光滑,其象当毛,毛无芒刺,必得淡红上有薄白之胎气,方是无邪之舌"。又说"舌色淡红,平人之常候……红者心之气,淡者胃之气"。《舌鉴总论》说:"舌乃心苗,心属火,其色赤,心居肺内,肺属金,其色白,故当舌质淡红,舌苔微白,而红必红润内充,白必苔微不厚,或略厚有花。然皆干湿得中,不滑不燥,斯为无病之舌,乃火藏金内之象"。《伤寒论本旨·辨舌苔》认为"舌苔由胃中生气所现,而胃气由心脾发生。故无病之人常有薄苔,是胃中之生气,如地上之微草也"。说明正常舌象的形成,与脏腑功能的正常活动有密切的关系,正常舌象是胃气旺盛、气血安和、脏腑功能正常的表现。

As to the mechanism of normal tongue picture, *Tongue Coating General Records* saying, "The tongue is the sprout of heat, the color is red, the texture is moist, the feature is fur-like without prickle, and all these manifestations should contribute embryo. Only this kind of tongue is regarded as normal tongue." Another saying, "Prink is normal color, red belongs to the heart and light belongs to *stomach-qi*." *General Records for Tongue Diagnosis* had pointed out, "The tongue is sprout of the heart, and the heart belongs to fire. Its color is red and it's located in thorax, the lung belongs to gold and its color is white. It's why the tongue texture is prinked while coating is white. By the way, the red includes red and moist, and the white refers to thin coating, also refers to thick and moderate coating sometimes. It is manifestation of gold-hidden fire." *Coating Diagnosis*, one of Chapter in *Sprit of Treatise on Cold-Attack* states, "The tongue coating is produced by steaming *stomach-qi*, which is commanded by the heart and spleen." So in healthy body, there is a little thin coating like grass roots. It is the embodiment of *stomach-qi* activity. It is also suggested that the tongue is closely related to the normal function of viscera. In sum, normal tongue is embodiment of the exuberance of *stomach-qi*, the harmony of *qi* and blood, and the health of viscera.

3. 舌象的生理变异
3. Physiological change of Tongue

正常舌象受内外环境的影响,可以产生相应的生理性变异。因此,在掌握基本标准的前提下,还要注意某些生理变异,临床才能准确地判断舌象。

With internal and external environment changing, tongue will change accordingly, too. Thus, It's necessary to understand some physiological changes of tongue in clinic diagnosis.

(1) 年龄、性别因素
(1) Age and Sex

年龄是舌象产生生理性变异的因素之一,由于年龄的差异,舌象也会相应变异。如儿童阴阳幼稚之体,脾胃功能尚薄,处于生长发育快而营养相对不足的状态,故舌质多偏淡嫩(图 1.3.3.1),舌苔偏少易剥;老年人脏腑精气渐衰,气血多偏虚而运行较迟缓,故舌色偏暗红(图 1.3.3.2)。

The age is one of the factors of tongue change. As people have different ages, the tongue can change accordingly too. For example, young children have "tender yin" or "tender yang" constitution, and their spleen and stomach function have not still developed completely, what's more, they are growing up and those necessary nutriments

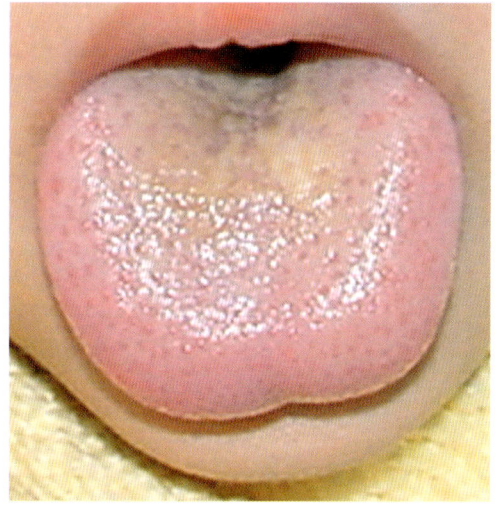

图(See color fig)1.3.3.1

acquired from food is in comparative shortage. All these factors lead to their tongue texture tends to be light and tender (See color fig. 1.3.3.1). Aged people because they have weak constitution accompanied by the insufficiency of *qi* and blood, and weakness of primordial *yin* and *yang*, the tongue color tends to dark red (See color fig. 1.3.3.2).

性别与舌象在一般情况下无显著差异,但女性因月经周期的生理影响,会出现经期舌蕈状乳头充血、舌质偏红、舌尖边部点刺增大,而经后则自行消退的现象(图 1.3.3.3)。

Generally speaking, sex has no obvious effect on tongue, but mature woman is special, because menses is unique physiological phenomenon for them. With menses appearing, the fungiform papillae congested, the color tends to red and the pickles enlarged on tongue tip. After menses, all these phenomena will disappear away naturally (See color fig. 1.3.3.3).

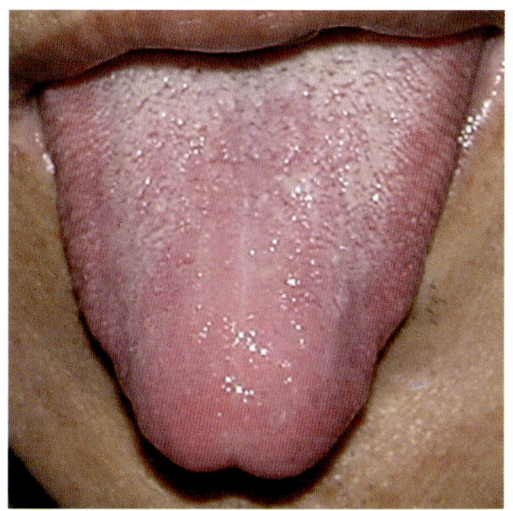

图(See color fig)1.3.3.2

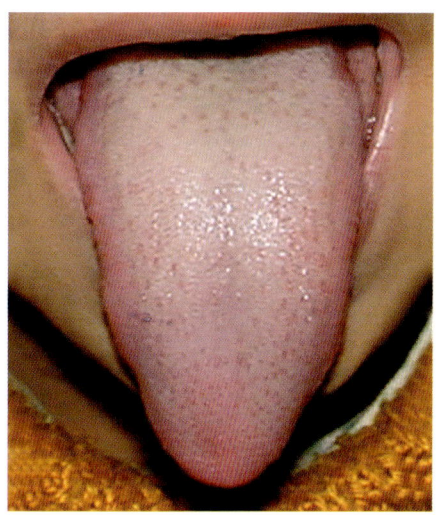

图(See color fig)1.3.3.3

（2）体质禀赋因素

(2) Constitution and Congenital Disposition

由于先天禀赋有不同,体质有差异,舌象亦可有变异,正如《辨舌指南》指出:"无病之舌,形舌各有不同,有常清洁者,有稍生苔层者,有鲜红者,有淡白色者,或为紧而尖,或为松而软,并有牙印着,此因无病时,各有享赋不同,故舌质亦异也。"如肥胖之人舌多胖大色淡(图1.3.3.4),消瘦之人舌多偏瘦色红(图1.3.3.5)。

People have different congenital disposition and constitution. So their tongues may be different accordingly. Just like *Guides for Tongue Diagnosis* points out, "As normal the tongue is, its texture nay be different, such as clear coating, a little coating, bright red, and light white coating, tense and sharp texture, loose and soft texture, even teeth-print texture. All these phenomena are caused by constitution and congenital disposition." That also can explain why fat peoples' tongue is mostly corpulence and light (See color fig. 1.3.3.4), while these thin peoples are mostly thin and red (See color fig. 1.3.3.5).

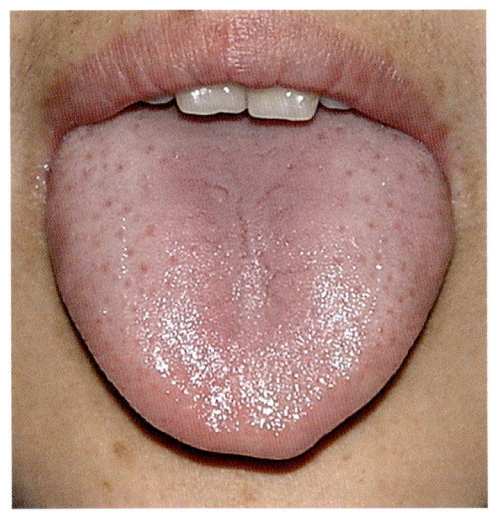
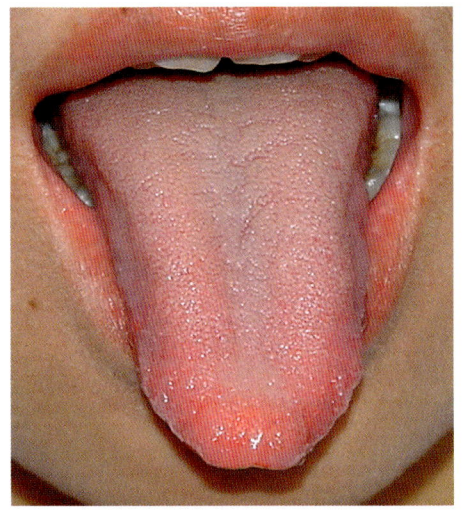

图(See color fig)1.3.3.4　　　　　　　图(See color fig)1.3.3.5

另外,先天性裂纹舌(图1.3.3.6)、齿痕舌(图1.3.3.7)、地图舌(图1.3.3.8)等,多见于禀赋不足、体质单薄者。他们虽可长期无明显临床病证,但具有对某些病因的易感性和病种的好发倾向,并影响疾病的转归与预后。

In addition, some abnormal tongue, like crack tongue (See color fig. 1.3.3.6) teeth-print tongue(See color fig. 1.3.3.7) and geographic tongue (See color fig. 1.3.3.8)are mostly formed because of shortage of congenital disposition and week constitutions. Although there is no syndrome in clinic, they have some potential factor to some pathogenesis and diseases, which influences prognosis of disease.

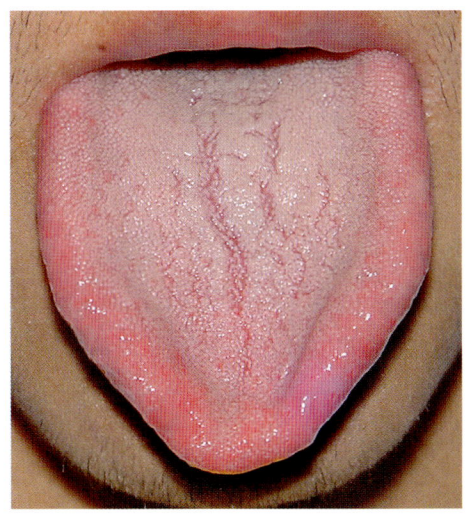
图(See color fig)1.3.3.6

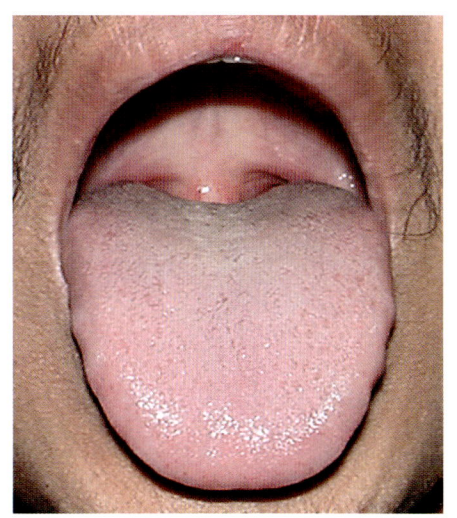
图(See color fig)1.3.3.7

(3) 气候环境因素
(3) Climate and Environment

季节与地域的差别会产生气候环境的变化,引起舌象相应变化。如《辨舌指南·辨舌质生苔之原理》指出:"平人舌中常有浮白苔一层,或浮黄苔一层,夏月湿土司令,苔每易较厚而微黄,但不满不滞",即夏季暑湿较盛,舌苔多易增厚,苔色多见淡黄(图1.3.3.9)。同理,秋季燥气当今,苔多偏薄偏干(图1.3.3.10);冬季严寒,舌常较湿润(图1.3.3.11)。

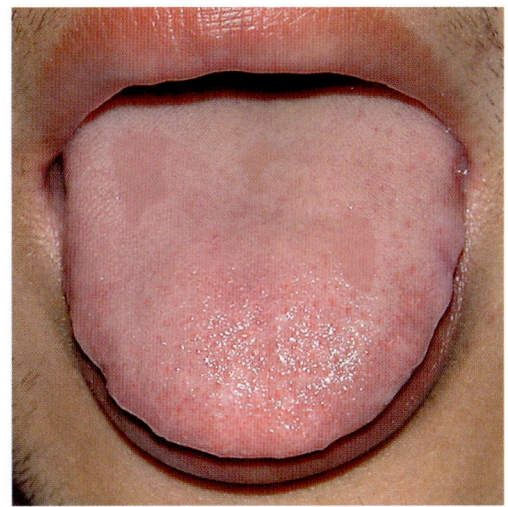
图(See color fig)1.3.3.8

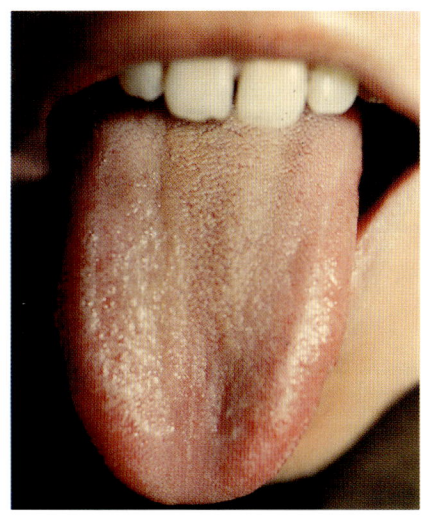
图(See color fig)1.3.3.9

People live and work in different regions and seasons, the tongue will change, too. As to the mechanism of tongue texture and coating, in *the Chapter of Guides for Tongue Diagnosis* says, "In the healthy body, there is a floating white coating, or floating yellow coating." The *dampness-qi* is active in summer, so it's easy to make the coating thick and slight yellow (See color fig. 1.3.3.9). Likewise, the *dryness-qi* is active in autumn, so the coating tends to thinness and dryness (See color fig. 1.3.3.10). Cold is active in winter and the coating is moist usually (See color fig. 1.3.3.11).

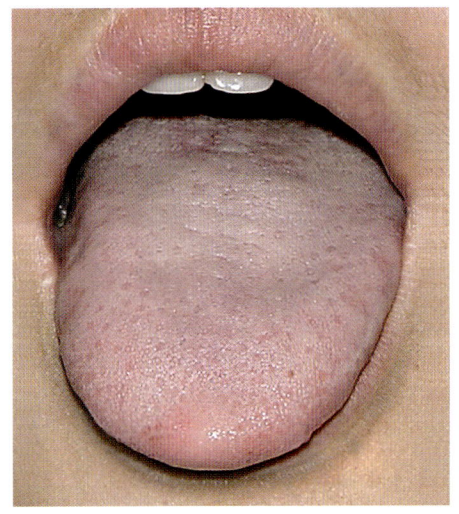 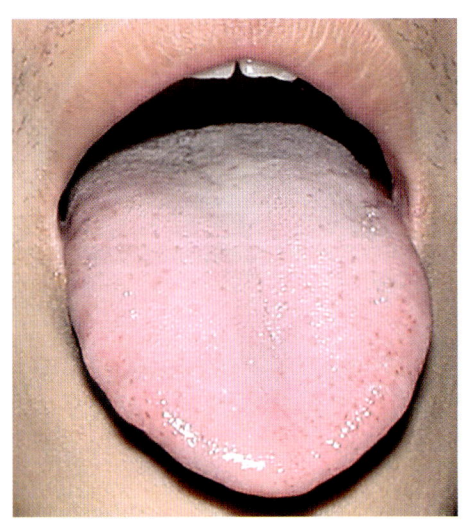

图(See color fig) 1.3.3.10　　　　　　　图(See color fig)1.3.3.11

我国东南地区偏湿偏热、西北与东北地区寒冷干燥的地理差异,也会使舌象产生类似的影响。这些都是人体生理活动与自然环境息息相应在舌象上的反映。

In southeast of China, climate is damp and hot, on the contrary, climate is cold and dry in northwest and northeast of China, and these factors change tongue correspondingly. It also is a reflection of relationship between the natural world and the human being.

(4) 生活起居习性因素
(4) Habits and Customs

一日之间,饮食起居变化也会影响舌象。如晨起之际,舌苔相对较厚(图1.3.3.12)、进食之后,舌苔相对较薄(图1.3.3.13);体力活动之后,舌色可更红活(图1.3.3.14)。《辨舌指南·绪言》曰:"常人一日三餐,故苔亦三变,谓之活苔,无病之象"。

Diet and habit can change tongue. For example, tongue coating is thicker in the morning (See color fig. 1.3.3.12) and thin after food (See color fig. 1.3.3.13). Taking part in labor physical activities promotes the circulation of *qi* and blood, so the tongue color becomes more red and brighter (See color fig. 1.3.3.14). *Preface of Guides for Tongue Diagnosis* states, "People have meal for 3 times every day, the coating changes for 3 times, too. Only this kind of coating is regarded as lively coating, of cause, it is beyond disease."

日常生活中的习惯及饮食嗜好,对舌象会造成干扰。如嗜烟者,苔易发褐(图1.3.3.15);嗜酒者,苔易黄腻(图1.3.3.16);嗜茶者,舌多湿润(图1.3.3.17);张口呼吸,舌易发干(图1.3.3.18);习惯刮舌,厚苔变薄(图1.3.3.19);禁食较久,苔会累积变厚等(图.1.3.3.20)。

Habits in daily life and hobbies of drink and food may disturb the express of the tongue. For example, a person who has a liking for smoking usually has a brown tongue (See color fig. 1.3.3.15), and a person being addicted to drink always has a yellow and greasy fur (See color fig. 1.3.3.16), but a person who favorites tea often has a moist tongue (See color fig. 1.3.3.17). The tongue may be dried because of breathing with mouth open (See color fig. 1.3.3.18), thick fur will turn to thin for the habit of scraping the tongue (See color fig. 1.3.3.19). Food forbidden for a long time may thicken the fur (See color fig. 1.3.3.20).

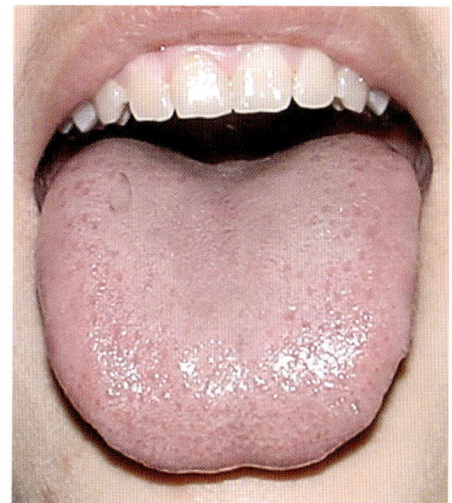

图(See color fig)1.3.3.12

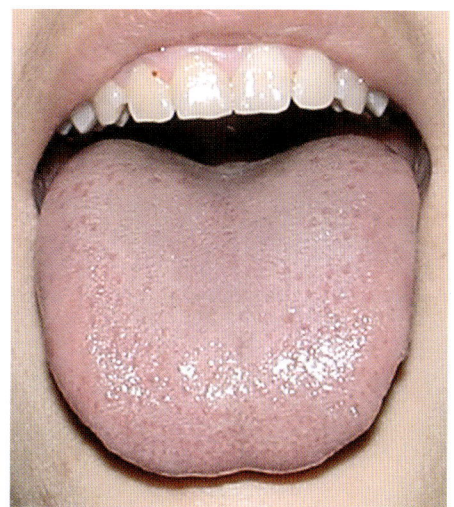

图(See color fig)1.3.3.13

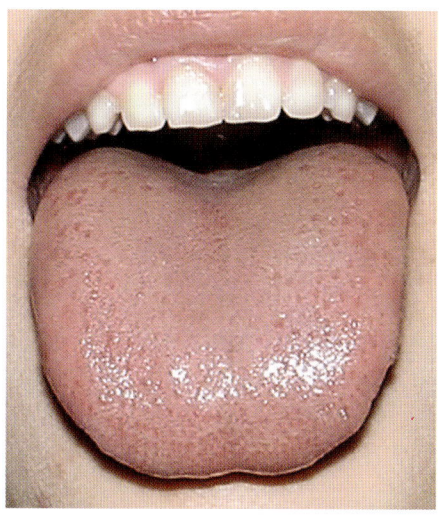

图(See color fig)1.3.3.14

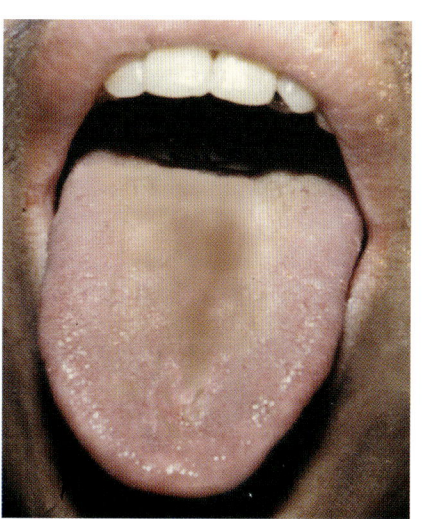

图(See color fig)1.3.3.15

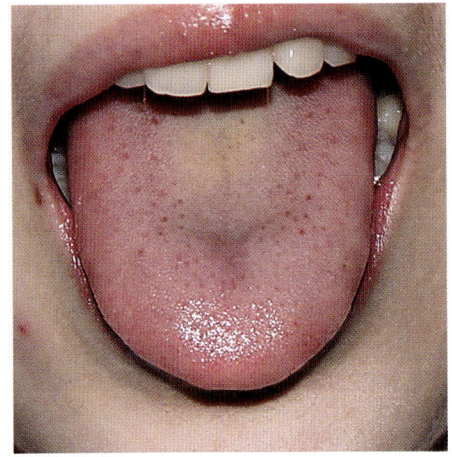
图(See color fig)1.3.3.16

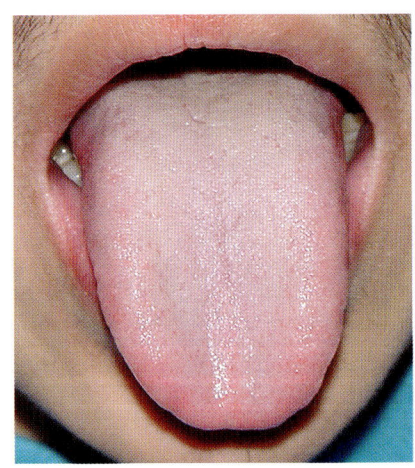
图(See color fig)1.3.3.17

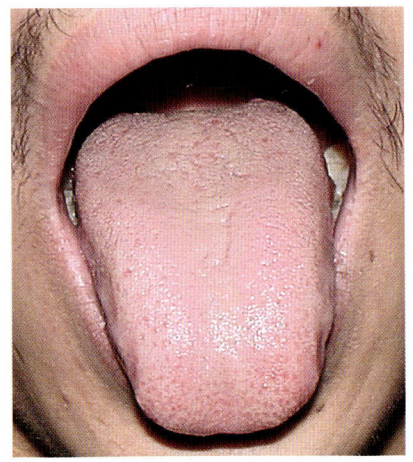
图(See color fig)1.3.3.18

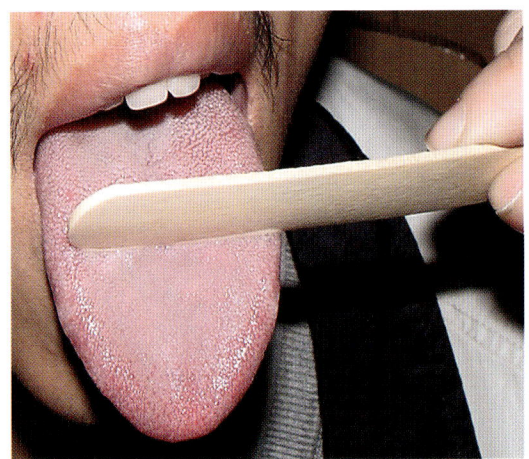
图(See color fig.)1.3.3.19

此外,值得注意的是,正常人出现异常舌象,除了上述生理因素外,有一部分可能是潜在疾病的前期征象,由于舌象能迅速灵敏地反映机体内部的病变,即有些内在的病变,通过舌象的灵敏变化,会先于自觉症状而表现出来。因此,临床实践中发现平常人有异常舌象时,首先要结合问诊,慎重鉴别,认真分析,看其是真正的生理变异还是舌先于症状的潜伏病态。必要时进行随访观察。

It is notable that normal people who may have an abnormal tongue sometimes, which may be an early stage expression of potential disease besides physiological cause as the above. Since the tongue can reflect the pathological changes of the interior quickly and sensitively, a person has interior pathological changes whose tongue will be acutely changed before the ap-

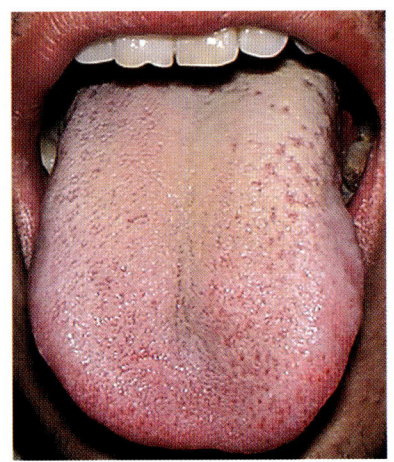
图(See color fig)1.3.3.20

pearance of conscious syndromes. So, when we find a normal person having abnormal tongue during our clinical practice, we should study which in the light of inquisition at first, then distinguish which is due to the true physiological changes or is due to the potential disease, and we must call on and watch the person at the necessary time.

第二章 诊舌质

Chapter Two Observation of the tongue texture

舌质又称舌体,是舌的肌肉和脉络组织,诊舌质主要观察舌神、舌色、舌形、舌态和舌下脉络等内容。

The tongue texture or the tongue body consists of muscles, vessels, channels and collaterals in the tongue. Observing tongue texture is to observe the vitality, color, shape, movement of the tongue body and the channels and collaterals under the tongue.

第一节 诊舌神
Section 1　Observations of the tongue vitality

舌神,即舌之神气,是人体生命活动在舌上的集中表现。通过观察舌神的有无,可从总体上把握体内脏腑精气之盛衰、机体生机之胜败、疾病转归之凶吉等基本状况。《望诊遵经·望舌诊法提纲》指出:"神也者,……得之则生,失之则死,变化不可离,斯须不可去者也"。

The Tongue vitality, or the expression of the tongue, centralizes the expression of the body life. Thus, observing the tongue vitality we can learn the condition of vital essence of the zang-fu organs, the depth of the location of illness and the severity of disease. As *Classic Observation Outline of Tongue Observation* say, "A person having vitality can exist for a long time while a person lacking of vitality may be dying".

舌神的基本特征主要表现在舌体的色泽与动态两方面。

The tongue vitality is shown in color and mobility of tongue texture.

1. 有神
1. Full vitality

舌体红活明润、运动灵活者为有神(图 2.1.1.1),舌体有神,说明阴阳气血精神皆足、富有生机,虽病亦属善候,预后较好。

Full vitality tongue means that a light red tongue body with energetic movement and enough fluid of it (See color fig. 2.1.1.1). It suggests plentiful *qi*, blood, *Yin*, *Yang* and spirit, and the prognosis are good.

2. 无神
2. Lacking of vitality (out of vitality)

舌体晦黯枯萎、呆板僵滞者为无神(图 2.1.2.1)。舌体无神,说明阴阳气血精神皆败、生机已微,预后较差。

The tongue lacking of vitality refers to dark and dry tongue body with sluggish movement (See color fig. 2.1.2.1). It suggests exhausting of *qi*, blood, *Yin*, *Yang* and spirit, and the prognosis is bad in this condition.

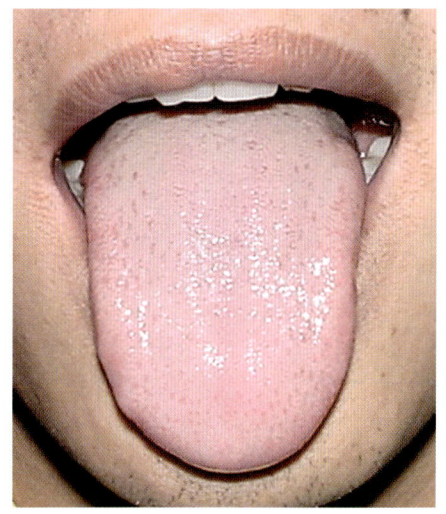
图(See color fig)2.1.1.1

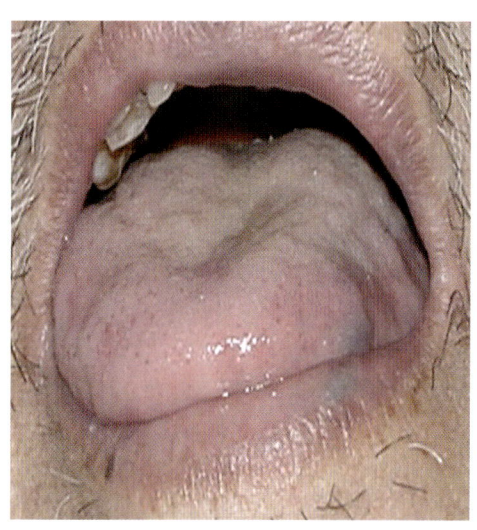
图(See color fig)2.1.2.1

《辨舌指南·辨舌之神气》曰:"荣者,有光彩也,凡病皆吉;枯者,无精神也,凡病皆凶。荣润则津足,干枯则津乏。荣者为有神……明润而有血色者生,枯暗而无血色者死。凡舌质有光有体,不论黄白灰黑,刮之而里面红润,神气荣华者,诸病皆吉;若舌质无光无体,不拘有苔无苔,视之里面枯晦,神气全无者,诸病皆凶。"可见,舌神之有无,反映了脏腑、气血、津液之盛衰,关系到疾病预后之吉凶。

Guides for Tongue Diagnosis · Distinguishing the Tongue Vitality say, "The flourish of tongue means the tongue has luster and the prognosis is good. The withering is out of vitality and the prognosis is bad. The flourish of tongue refers to enough fluid on it while the withering refers to exhausting fluid on it. The flourish means full of vitality, it suggest that a person having plentiful of blood and he will exist for a long time. The withering suggested the lacking of blood of the body that will be dying. If the condition is red, moist and vigorous, no matter the color of tongue coating is yellow, white or black, the prognosis is good. If the condition is dark and dry, no matter there is coating or not, the prognosis is very bad."

第二节 诊 舌 色
Section Two Observations of The Tongue Color

舌体的颜色可分为淡红、淡白、红色、绛色、紫色、青色等几种,除淡红色为正常舌色之外,其余颜色均属于病色。

There are pink, pale white, red, crimson, purplish and blue colors of tongue. Pink is the normal color of tongue body and the other colors are the abnormal color.

1. 淡红舌
1. The Pink Tongue

舌色淡红润泽,不浅不深。为心血充足,胃气旺盛,气血调和之征象,常见于健康人(图2.2.1.1)。

Pink is the normal color of tongue body. The normal condition is neither too light nor too deep pink color of whole tongue body. It suggests sufficient heart blood and vigorous stomach *qi*. It means reconciliation of *qi* and blood (See color fig. 2.2.1.1).

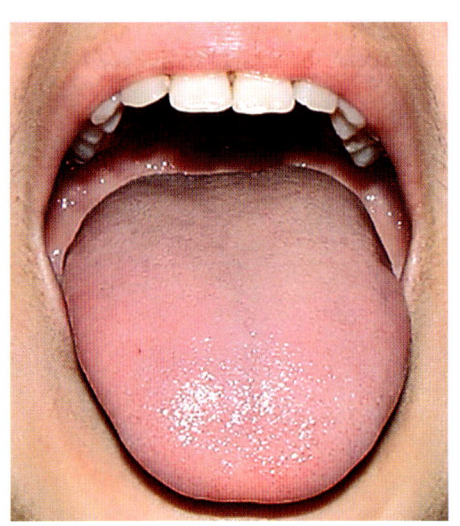

图(See color fig)2.2.1.1

淡红为舌体之本色,《舌苔统志·淡红舌》说:"舌色淡红,平人之候……红者心之气,淡者胃之气。"《舌鉴辨证·红舌总论》亦说:"全舌淡红,不浅不深者,平人也。"

Tongue Coating General Records • *Pink Tongue* refer,"The pink is normal color of the tongue body. The red tongue comes from h*eart qi* and the pale comes from *stomach qi*. *Syndrome Differentiation on Tongue general discussion for red tongue refers*,"Pink is the normal color of the tongue body, which is neither too light nor too deep, and usually can be seen from a healthy person."

在外感病初期,舌色淡红,为外邪侵犯肌表,尚未侵及气血与脏腑,属病情轻浅。

A pink tongue in the early period of the exogenous diseases suggests that the disease is in the exterior and not in *qi*, blood and *zang-fu*, and the state of illness is light.

2. 淡白舌
2. The Pale Tongue

舌色比正常舌色浅淡,红色偏少而白色偏多,称为淡白舌。多因气血亏虚,血不荣舌,或阳气虚衰,运血无力,舌失血充,致舌色浅淡。

A tongue which color is light than that of normal is known as pale tongue, which shows less red and much more white color. It is due to decline of *qi* and *yang*, or blood deficiency. The deficient *yang* and *qi* fails to send blood up to the tongue, and the deficient blood fails to nourish the tongue, so the color becomes pale.

舌色淡白而舌体瘦小,多为气血两虚,血不上荣(图 2.2.2.1.);若舌色淡白,几无血色,干枯少津,则称为枯白舌。多为阳虚不能运血、或脱血夺气,气血失充(图 2.2.2.2);若舌色淡白,舌体胖极,舌边有齿印,舌面湿润多津者,多为阳虚水湿内停(图 2.2.2.3);若舌色淡白,舌面光滑无苔,则称为淡白光莹舌。为脾胃之气衰败,气血衰败之候(图 2.2.2.4)。

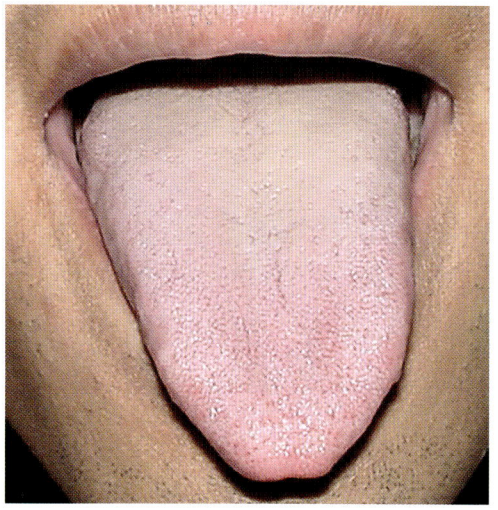

In general, the pale tongue with an emaciated body suggests the deficiency of both *qi* and blood, and the deficient blood failing to nourish the tongue (See color fig. 2.2.2.1). While the pale tongue with less red color and fluid named as withered pale tongue, suggests the deficiency

图(See color fig)2.2.2.1

yang, which fails to carry blood, or the depletion of *qi* and blood which fails to nourish the tongue (See color fig. 2.2.2.2). The pale tongue with the fattest body and teeth-print and much fluid on coating implies deficiency of *yang* and water-dampness detention (See color fig. 2.2.2.3). While a pale slippery tongue without coating, which is called a pale transparent tongue, suggest exhaustion of *qi* and blood, and extremely deficient *qi* of spleen and stomach (See color fig. 2.2.2.4).

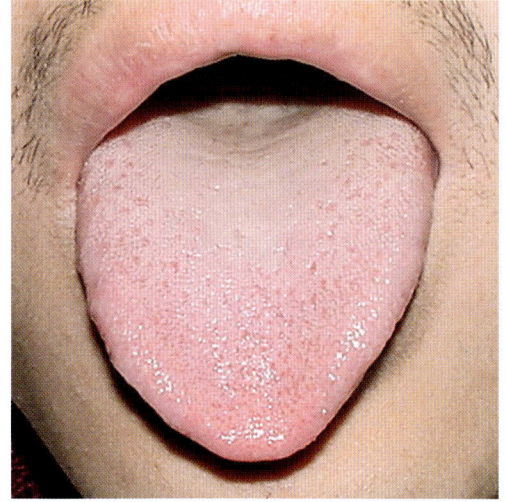

图(See color fig)2.2.2.2

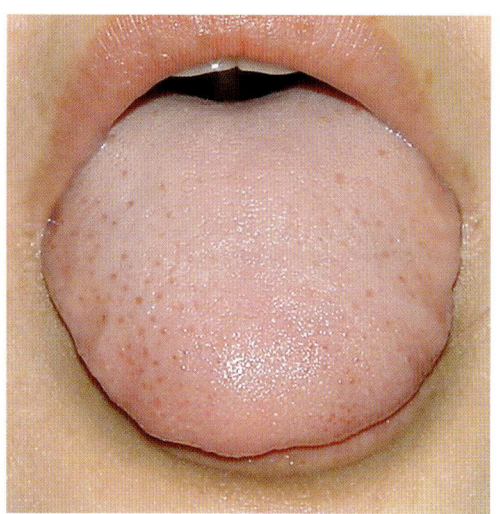

图(See color fig)2.2.2.3

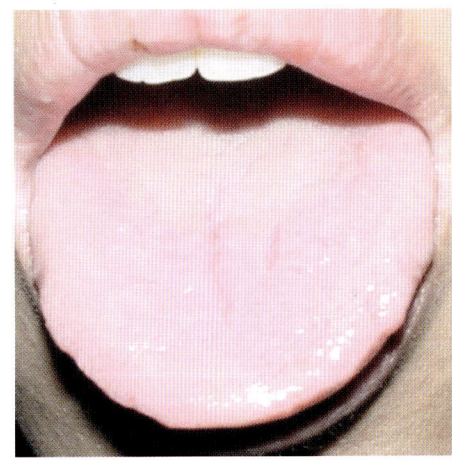

图(See color fig)2.2.2.4

3. 红舌
3. The Red Tongue

舌色较淡红颜色为深,呈鲜红色,主热证。因血得热则行,热盛则气血沸涌,舌体脉络充盈,或阴液亏虚,虚火上炎,故舌呈鲜红色。

When the red color of tongue is heavier than that of normal condition, it is called a red tongue. It suggests internal heat. Heat in body makes *qi* and blood boiling. Then the vessels of tongue are filled up. A red tongue is also resulted from upward invasion of asthenia heat as a result of deficiency of *yin* and fluid.

舌边尖红,多为外感风热表证初期(图2.2.3.1);若舌色红,舌尖有芒刺,舌面兼黄厚苔者,多属实热证,在外感病中出现多为热盛期(图2.2.3.2),在内伤病见之为脏腑阳热亢盛(图2.2.3.3);若舌色红而干,舌面少苔或无苔,或有裂纹者,多为阴虚火旺(图2.2.3.4);若舌色红,舌苔黄腻者,多属湿热证(图2.2.3.5);若舌色红,舌苔白如积粉者,多因外感秽浊湿邪与热毒相结而成(图2.2.3.6);舌尖独红,为心火上炎(图2.2.3.7);舌边红赤,为肝胆有热(图2.2.3.8);舌红中剥,为胃阴已伤(图2.2.3.9);舌红瘦薄而干燥,为热盛津伤(图2.2.3.10)。

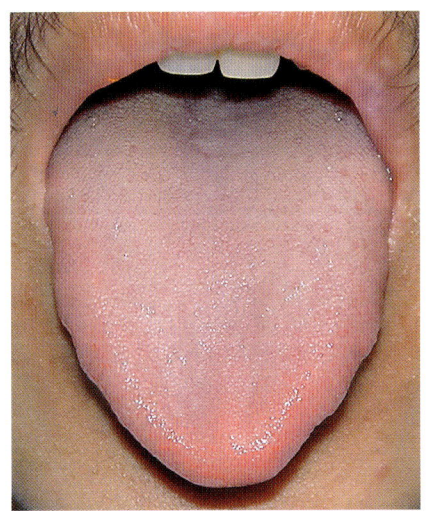

图(See color fig)2.2.3.1

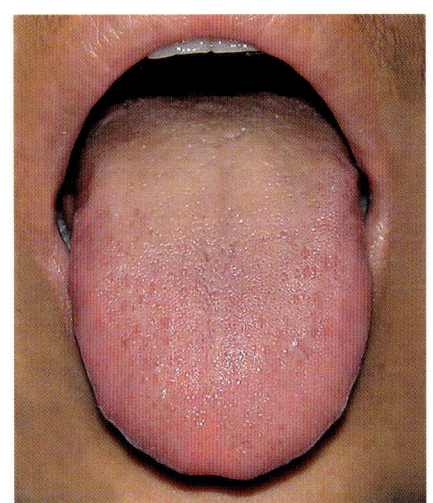

图(See color fig)2.2.3.2

The red margin and tip of the tongue is caused by the exogenous wind-heat (See color fig. 2.2.3.1). The bright red tongue with rough and prickly fur, or with thick and yellowish fur mostly suggests excess-heat syndrome (See color fig. 2.2.3.2); It suggests extreme heat during the exogenous disease period and excessive heat of *yang* and *zang-fu* during the endogenous injury period (See color fig. 2.2.3.3); A withered red tongue with less coating or without any coating or with crack on the body mostly results from upward invasion of asthenia heat as a result of deficiency of *yin* (See color fig. 2.2.3.4); A red tongue with yellow greasy coating usually suggest heat with dampness (See color fig. 2.2.3.5). A red tongue with white coating like piled flour being due to the combination of exogenous turbid *qi* of dampness with heat evil (See color fig. 2.2.3.6). If the red color is only at the tongue tip, it is due to heart fire flaming up (See color fig. 2.2.3.7). The red tongue in bilateral margins dues to liver and gallbladder fire (See color fig. 2.2.3.8). Red tongue with exfoliated fur suggest the injury of stomach *yin* (See color fig. 2.2.3.9). While a red dry and thin tongue means the hurt of fluid due to the excessive heat (See color fig. 2.2.3.10).

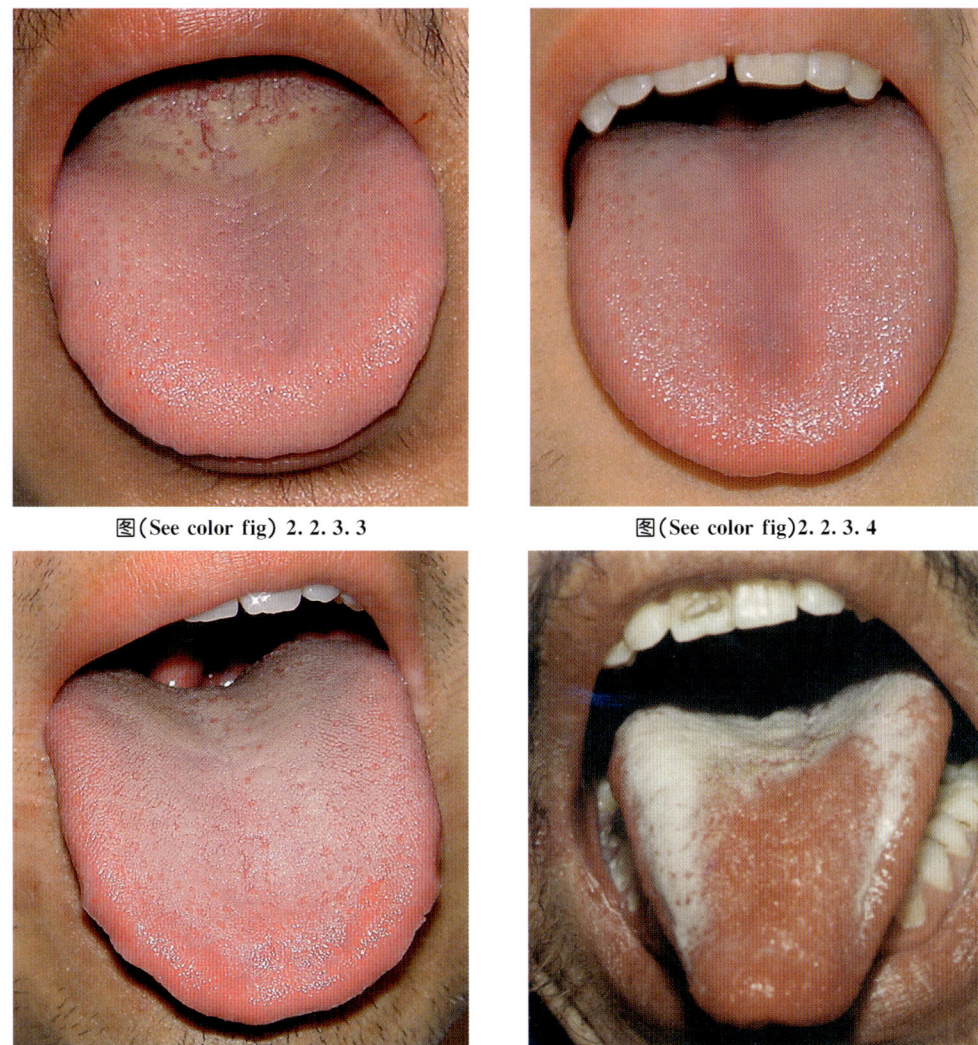

图(See color fig) 2.2.3.3　　　　　　　图(See color fig)2.2.3.4

图(See color fig)2.2.3.5　　　　　　　图(See color fig)2.2.3.6

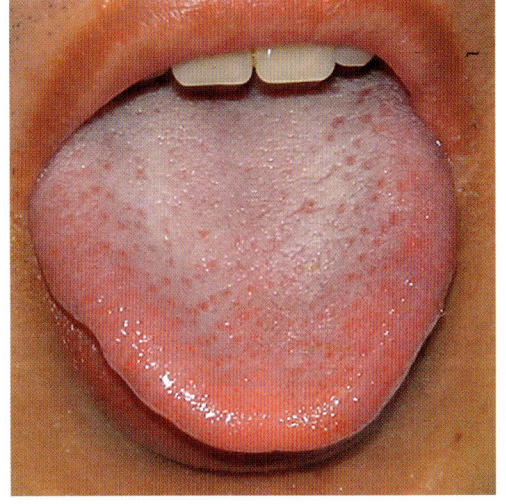
图(See color fig)2.2.3.7

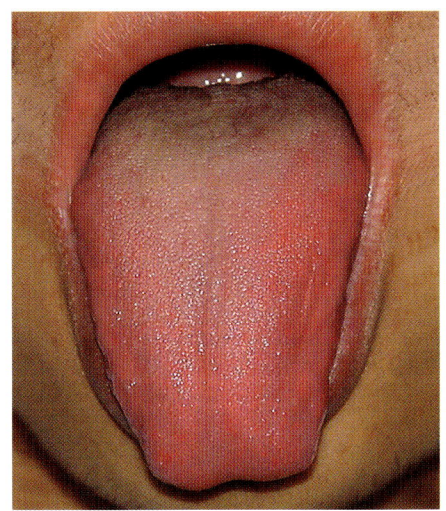
图(See color fig)2.2.3.8

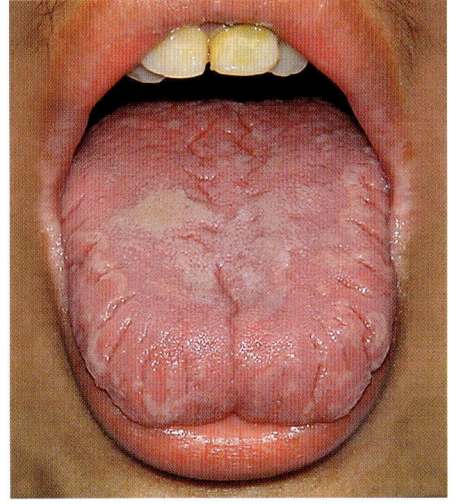
图(See color fig)2.2.3.9

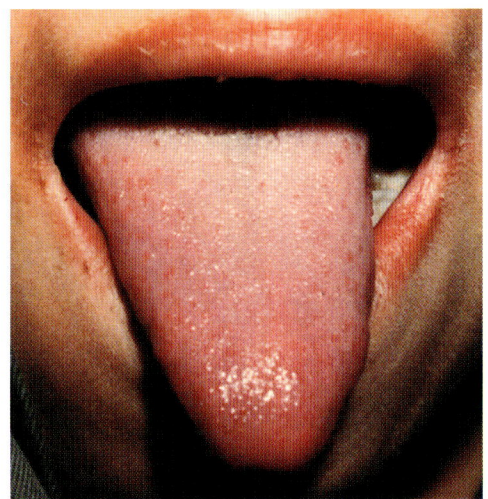
图(See color fig)2.2.3.10

《舌鉴辨证·红舌总论》指出:"表里虚实寒热证皆有红舌,赤红为脏腑具热,紫红瘀红为脏腑热极,多见于时疫或误服温补,鲜红无苔无津为阴虚火炎,色灼红无苔而燥干者为阴虚水涸"。

Syndrome Differentiation on Tongue · Red Tongue, a especially book on tongue, say, "The red tongue can been seen in exterior, interior cold, heat, deficiency and excess syndromes. A bright red tongue suggests excessive heat of *zang-fu*. A purple red tongue means extremely heat of zang-fu because of seasonal diseases or wrongly using warm and recuperate. A bright red tongue without any fur results from upward invasion of asthenia heat being due to the deficiency of yin. A dry red tongue without coating suggests exhaustion of fluid and deficiency of *yin*."

4. 绛舌
4. The Crimson Tongue

绛为深红色,比红舌的颜色更深更浓,主热盛。绛舌多由红舌进一步发展而成,多因热入营血,耗伤营阴,血液浓缩或阴虚水涸,虚火上炎所致。

Crimson tongue comes from red tongue. The color is more heavier and darker than red. It is often seen in the stage of extreme fever. It is resulted from upward invasion of asthenias heat because of deficiency of yin and exhaustion of fluid, or the exhaustion of *yin* and *yin* hurted by the heat that results in blood concentrated.

舌绛在外感病中出现,为热邪侵入营血之征象,多见舌绛而干,或伴见芒刺(图 2.2.4.1.)、(图 2.2.4.2);《辨舌指南·辨舌之颜色》说:"绛色心经,候营分血分之温热也,凡邪热传营舌色必绛。"在内伤病中出现,为阴液亏虚,虚火亢盛之候,多见舌绛少苔或无苔,或有裂纹(图 2.2.4.3)、(图 2.2.4.4);若舌绛而光莹,为胃肾阴亏已竭(图 2.2.4.5)、(图 2.2.4.6)。

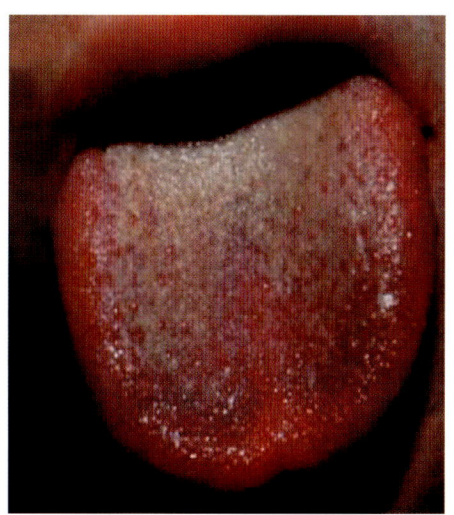 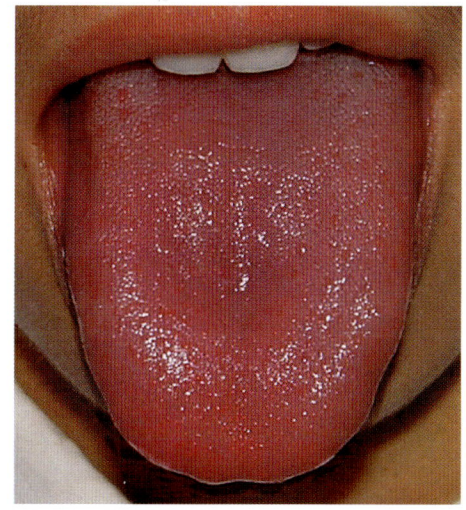

图(See color fig)2.2.4.1　　　　　　　　图(See color fig)2.2.4.2

A dry crimson tongue, or with prickles, which can be seen in the exogenous diseased, suggests invasion into *yin* and blood by heat evil (See color fig. 2.2.4.1), (See color fig. 2.2.4.2). *Guides for Tongue Diagnosis • Differentiation of the Tongue Color* says, "When heat entered nutrient-phase, the tongue color must be crimson, and the crimson tongue suggest warm-heat evil having entered into nutrient-phase and blood." A crimson tongue with less coating or no coating or with crack, which usually can be seen in the endogenous injury, suggests excessive asthenia heat resulting from deficiency of *yin* and fluid (See color fig. 2.2.4.3), (See color fig. 2.2.4.4). A crimson with transparent coating results from exhaustion of *yin* of stomach and kidney (See color fig. 2.2.4.5), (See color fig. 2.2.4.6).

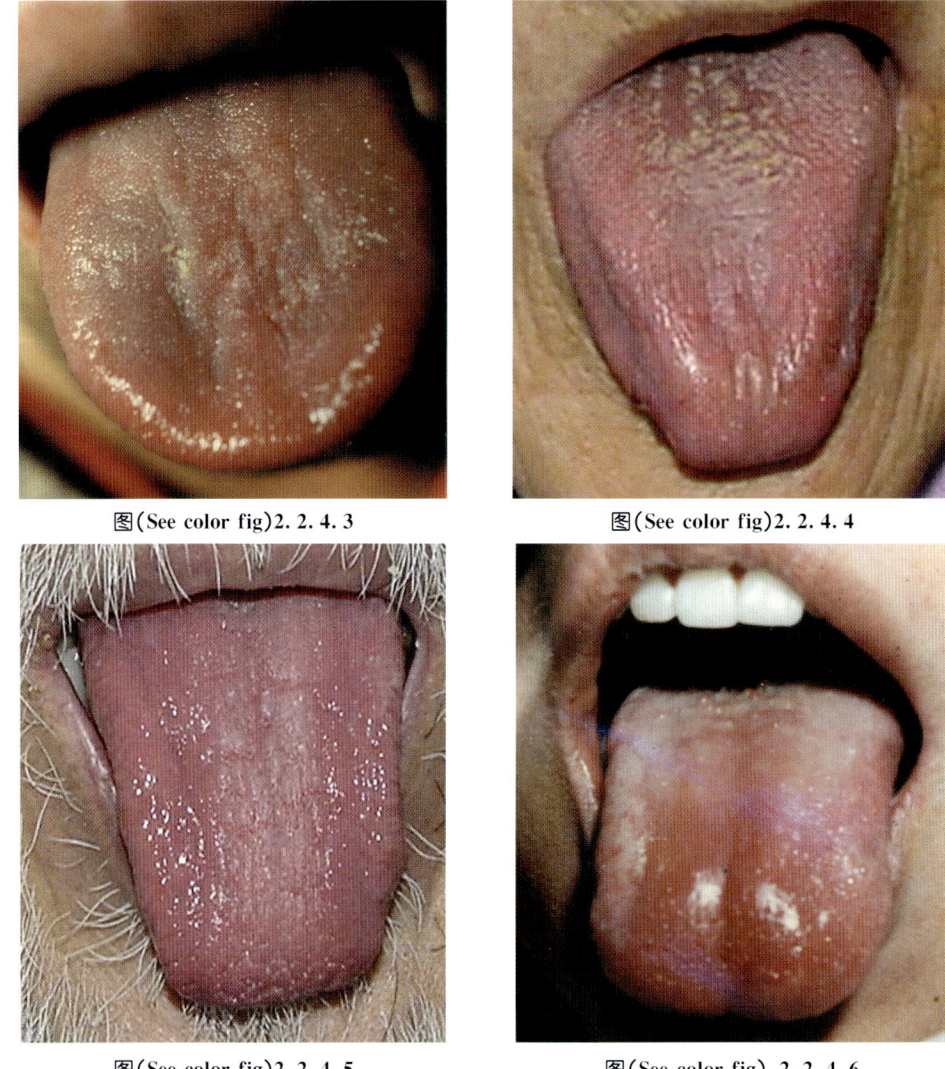

图(See color fig)2.2.4.3　　　　　　图(See color fig)2.2.4.4

图(See color fig)2.2.4.5　　　　　　图(See color fig).2.2.4.6

5. 紫舌
5. The Purple Tongue

　　舌淡紫、绛紫、青紫均称为紫舌。为气血运行不畅的病理改变。或因于寒、或因于热、或因于阳虚、或因于酒毒等，致血行不畅，瘀而为紫色。

　　A purplish tongue means that the tongue color is pale purple, crimson purple or blue purple. It is usually caused by the stagnation of *qi* and blood. Which results from cold, heat deficiency of heat or the injury by alcoholic toxin.

　　舌淡紫或青紫湿润主寒证；绛紫干枯少津主热证。舌色淡紫，或紫暗而湿润，多为阳虚寒盛,气血运行不畅之证(图 2.2.5.1);舌色绛紫,干枯少津,多为火热炽盛,营阴受损之证(图 2.2.5.2);舌绛紫舌肿大,多为酒毒冲心(图 2.2.5.3);舌色青紫,多为寒凝气滞,血液瘀阻之证(图 2.2.5.4);舌色青紫也可见于先天性心脏病,或药物、食物中毒等病证。

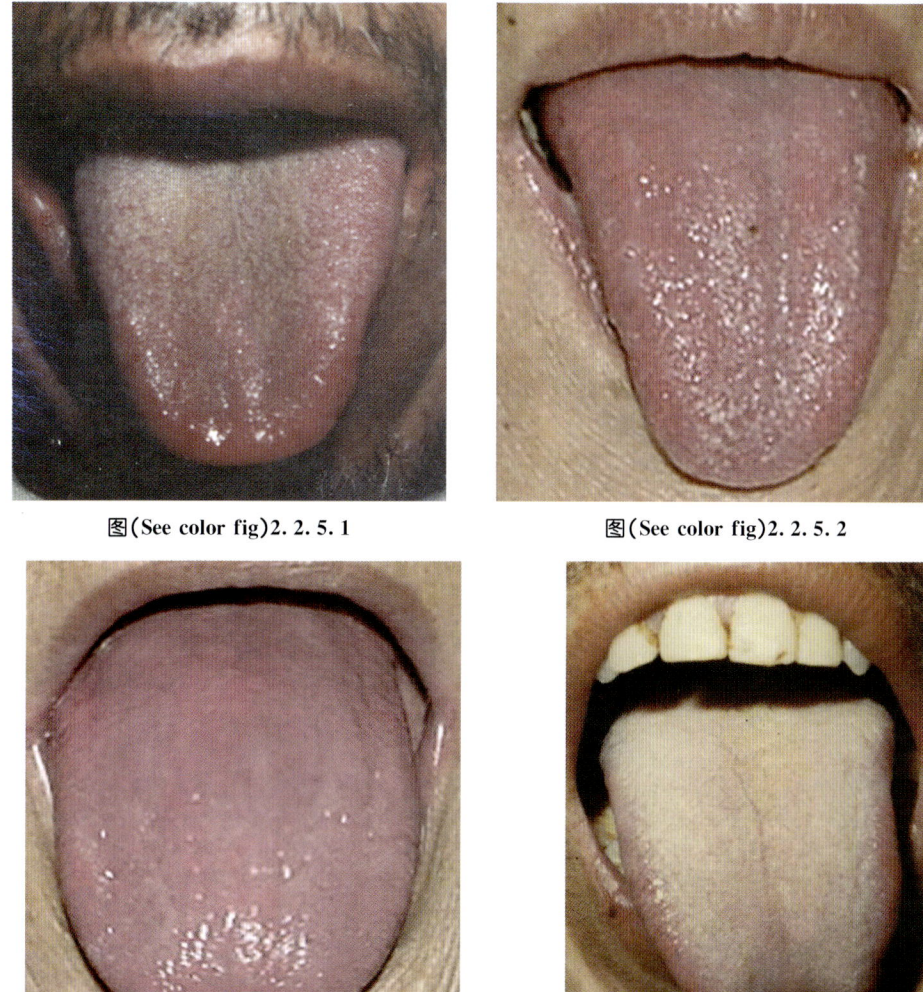

图(See color fig)2.2.5.1　　　　　　　图(See color fig)2.2.5.2

图(See color fig)2.2.5.3　　　　　　　图(See color fig)2.2.5.4

A pale or darken greasy purple tongue suggests coldness, while a withered crimson purple with less fluid suggests heat syndromes. The pale or darken greasy purple tongue mostly results from the stagnation of *qi* and blood caused by *yang* deficiency which fails to warm and push them in movement (See color fig. 2.2.5.1). The withered crimson purple tongue always dues to injury of nutrient-yin caused by excessive heat (See color fig. 2.2.5.2). The purple and swelling tongue is due to alcoholic toxin invading the heart (See color fig. 2.2.5.3). When the tongue body is light blue and purple, it is called bluish purple tongue. It is due to coagulated blood and stagnated *qi* by the coldness (See color fig. 2.2.5.4). A purple tongue also can be seen in congenital heart diseases, and the syndromes causing by toxin of foods and drugs.

6. 青舌
6. The Blue Tongue

舌色如皮肤暴露之"青筋",全无血色称为青舌。古人形容如同水牛之舌,多因寒凝阳郁、或阳虚寒凝、或瘀血停留所致。

When the tongue is blue without any red color it is called a blue tongue. In ancient time, it was called a "buffalo tongue". The blue tongue often indicates stagnations of *yang* by coldness, or deficiency of *yang* and combination of coldness, or the blood stasis.

全舌发青,是寒邪直中肝肾,阳气衰极或阳郁不宣所致(图2.2.6.1);舌边发青,是内有瘀血阻滞,血液运行不畅之故(图2.2.6.2)。

The whole blue tongue is due to direct cold attack of the liver and kidney, or the extremely different *yang*, or the stagnated *yang* (See color fig. 2.2.6.1). Blue in tongue margin is due to internal blood stasis (See color fig. 2.2.6.2).

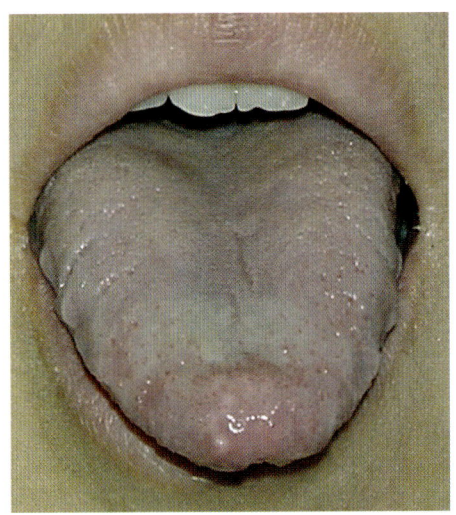 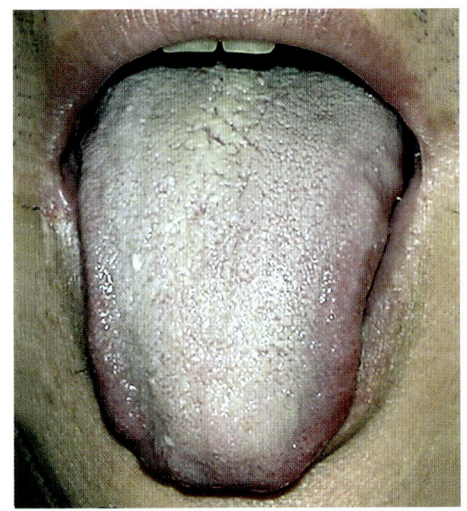

图(See color fig)2.2.6.1　　　　　　图(See color fig)2.2.6.2

《舌苔统志》认为:全舌青者,或口燥而漱水不欲咽,是内有瘀血。《辨舌指南》认为:肝属木,青色应肝,青舌候厥阴阴毒之危证。

Tongue Coating General Records considered that blue tongue with dry mouth difficulty of swallowing water but gargling is a sign of blood stasis. *Guides for Tongue Diagnosis* considered that liver belongs to wood, and the blue color indicates liver disease. So the blue tongue is sign of dangerous syndromes of the toxin of *JueYin*.

第三节 诊 舌 形
Section 3　Observation of the Tongue Shape

舌形是指舌质的形质,正常舌形,表现为柔软灵活,不大不小,荣润光泽。病理舌形包括苍老、娇嫩、胖大、瘦薄、芒刺、齿痕、裂纹等异常变化。

Tongue shape is the out figure of tongue body. The normal shape of the tongue is soft and flexible, neither too big nor too small, with gloss and moist. Its abnormal changes include tenderness, toughness, prickle, teeth-print, fissure and so on.

1. 苍老舌
1. The Tough Tongue

舌质纹理粗糙或皱缩,坚敛而不柔软,舌色较暗者,称为苍老舌(图 2.3.1.1)。多因实邪亢盛,充斥体内,而正气未衰,邪正交争,邪气壅滞于上所致。

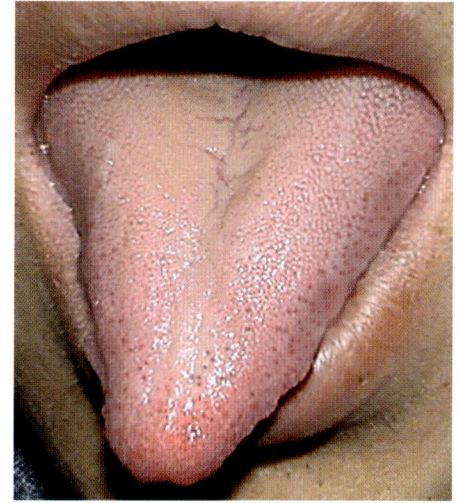

图(See color fig.)2.3.1.1

Striates of tongue are rough and sturdy which the color of tongue is dark (See color fig. 2.3.1.1). It results from excessive evil congesting in the body, with which underlining *genuine-qi* fight, and the stagnation in the *Upper-Jiao* because of the evil.

舌质坚敛苍老,不论舌色如何,病多属实。正如《辨舌指南》所说:"凡舌质坚敛而苍老,不论苔色黄灰黑,病多实证。"

The tough tongue, no matter what color of its body, mostly indicates excess syndromes. *Guides for Tongue Diagnosis* had said, "A rough and sturdy tongue, no matter with yellowish, gray or black coating, usually indicates excess syndrome.

2. 娇嫩舌
2. The Tender Tongue

舌体纹理细腻,浮胖娇嫩,舌色浅淡者,称为娇嫩舌(图 2.3.2.1)。多因气血不足,舌体脉络不充;或阳气亏虚,运血无力,舌体失养;或阳虚寒湿内生所致。

Striates of tongue are delicate, fine and smooth, and the color of the tongue is light (See color fig. 2.3.2.1). It results from deficient *qi* and blood falling to fill channels and collateral in the tongue, or deficient *yang* failing to carry blood to nourish the tongue body, or deficient *yang* resulting in retention of cold-dampness.

舌质浮胖娇嫩,无论舌色如何,多属虚证。正如《辨舌指南》所说:"凡舌质浮胖兼娇嫩,不拘苔色灰黑黄白,病多虚证。"

The tender tongue, no matter what color of its body, usually indicates deficiency syndromes. *Guides For Tongue Diagnosis* had said: "A tender tongue, no matter with gray, black yellowish or white coating, mostly indicates deficiency syndromes."

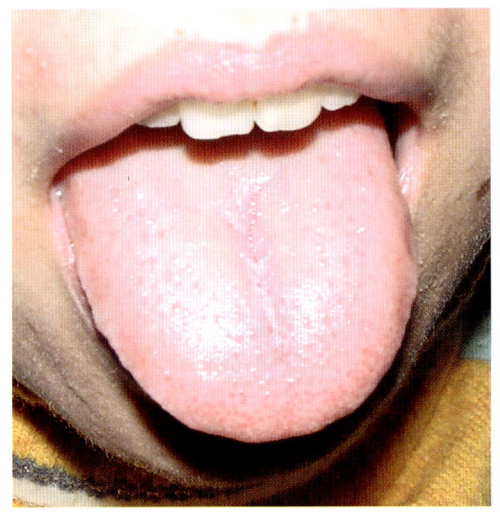

图(See color fig)2.3.2.1

3. 胖大舌
3. The Swelling Tongue

舌体较正常舌大而厚,伸舌满口,称为胖大舌(图2.3.3.1)。舌体肿大,伸舌盈口满嘴,甚则不能回缩,称为胖胀舌(图2.3.3.2)。多因水湿痰饮停滞,热毒、酒毒上犯所致。

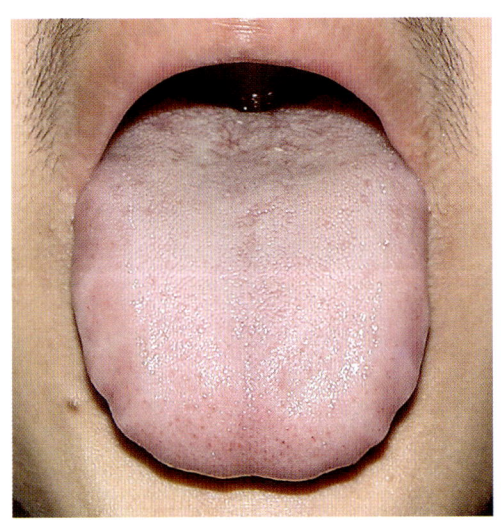

图(See color fig)2.3.3.1

The enlarged and swollen tongue body, even filling up mouth, is called a swollen tongue (See color fig. 2.3.3.1). The tongue body large in size, even filling up the whole mouth, or even failing to shrink back, is called a fat swollen tongue (See color fig. 2.3.3.2). It usually results from the stagnation of dampness and phlegm, or the invasion of heat-toxicity and alcoholic-toxicity.

舌体淡白胖大,舌面水滑,为脾肾阳虚,津液不化,水饮内停(图2.3.3.3);舌体红赤胖大,舌面有黄腻苔者,为脾胃湿热,或心胃热盛(图2.3.3.4);舌体绛紫肿大,为酒毒上冲,心火上炎(图2.3.3.5);舌紫暗胖大兼口唇发青,为中毒血瘀(图2.3.3.6)。

For example, the pale, puffy and tender tongue with moist fur is usually attributable to insufficiency of *spleen-yang* and *kidney-yang* and accumulation of the phlegm-damp (See color fig. 2.3.3.3). The red and corpulent tongue with yellow and greasy fur to damp-heat in the spleen and stomach, or excessive heat in the heart and stomach (See color fig. 2.3.3.4). The purplish and enlarged tongue, to upward attack of fire in the heart with alcoholic toxicity (See color fig. 2.3.3.5), and the puffy, bluish-purple and lusterless tongue, accompanying with blue lip, to stagnation of blood frequently seen in poisoning (See color fig. 2.3.3.6).

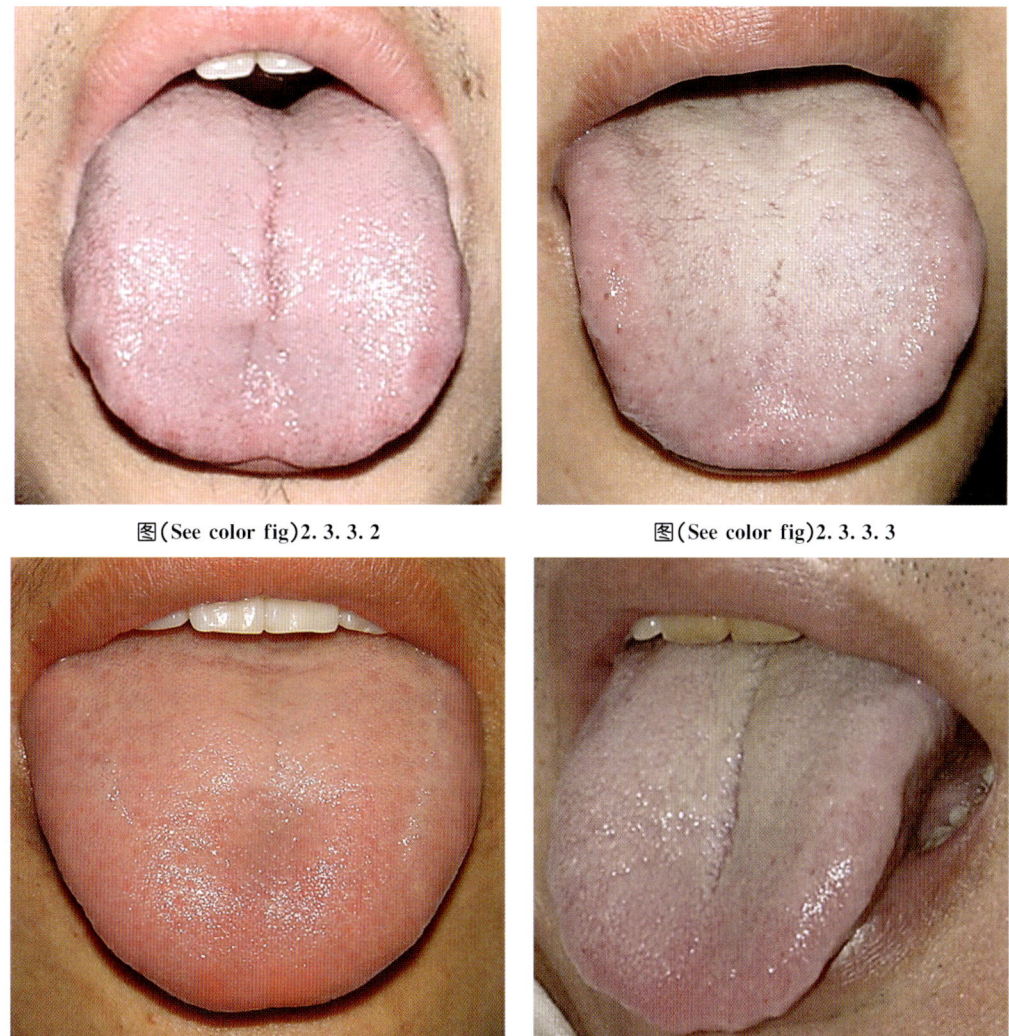

图(See color fig)2.3.3.2　　　　　　　图(See color fig)2.3.3.3

图(See color fig)2.3.3.4　　　　　　　图(See color fig)2.3.3.5

《辨舌指南·辨舌之形容》：说："舌赤胀大满口者,心胃之热也。舌赤肿满不得息者,心经热甚而血壅也。舌肿大者,或因热毒或因药毒也,唇舌紫暗青肿者,中毒也。舌紫肿厚者,酒毒上壅心火上炎也,或饮冷酒壅遏其热也。"

Guide For Tongue Diagnosis · shape and size of the tongue had said, "If the tongue body is swelling to fill up mouth, it is usually due to heat in the heart and stomach. The swollen tongue in red color mostly suggests excessive heat in heart channel and stagnation of blood. The swollen tongue in dark purple is often seen in alcohol poisoning or drug intoxication. The puffy, bluish-purple tongue and lip are frequently seen in poisoning. The thick, purplish and enlarged tongue often results from the upward attack of fire in the heart with alcoholic toxicity, or stagnation of heat caused by drinking cold alcohol."

4. 瘦薄舌
4. The Thin Tongue

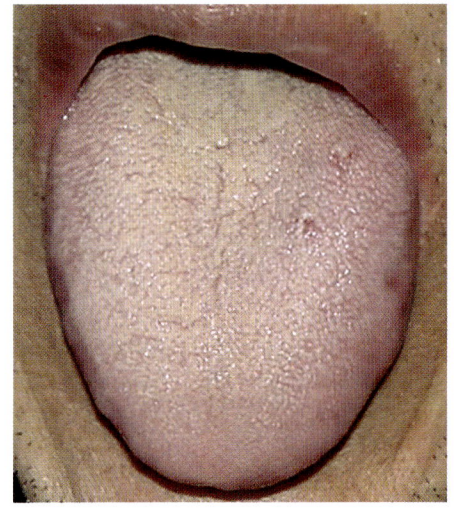

图(See color fig)2.3.3.6

舌体比正常瘦小而薄,称为瘦薄舌(图 2.3.4.1)。多因气血不足、不能充养舌体,舌体失养,或阴液亏虚,阴虚火旺所致。

A tongue smaller and thinner than normal in size is called thin tongue (See color fig. 2.3.4.1). It is usually caused by the deficient *qi* and blood failing to manifestation the tongue, or hyperactivity of fire due to deficiency of *yin* and fluid.

舌体淡白瘦薄,为气血两虚(图 2.3.4.2);舌体嫩红瘦薄,为心阴不足(图 2.3.4.3);舌体红绛瘦薄,为阴虚火旺(图 2.3.4.4)。

The pale thin tongue is usually due to *qi* and blood deficiency (See color fig. 2.3.4.2). The tender red thin tongue is usually due to insufficient *yin* in the heart (See color fig. 2.3.4.3); and the dry thin tongue in red or crimson is often due to fire flaring in yin deficiency (See color fig. 2.3.4.4).

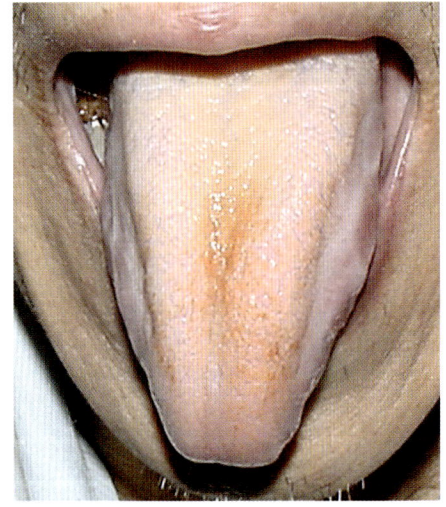

图(See color fig)2.3.4.1

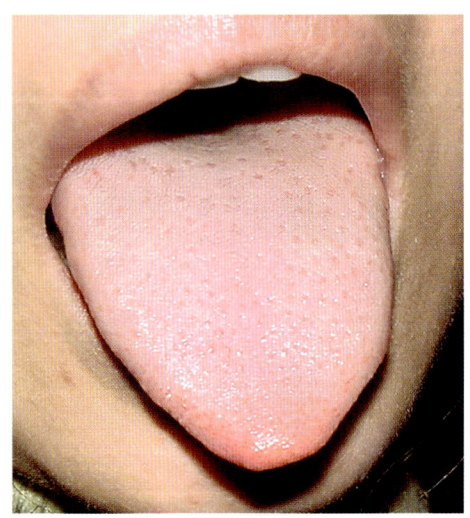

图(See color fig)2.3.4.2

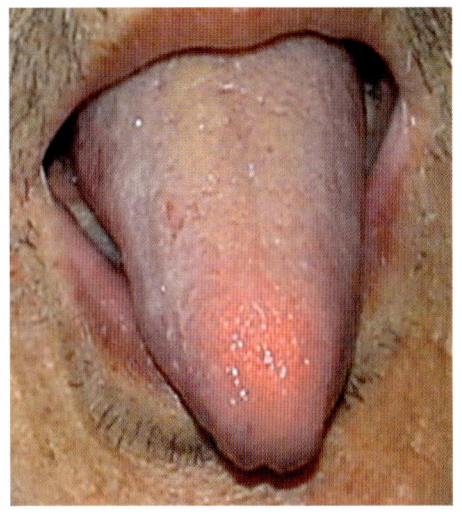 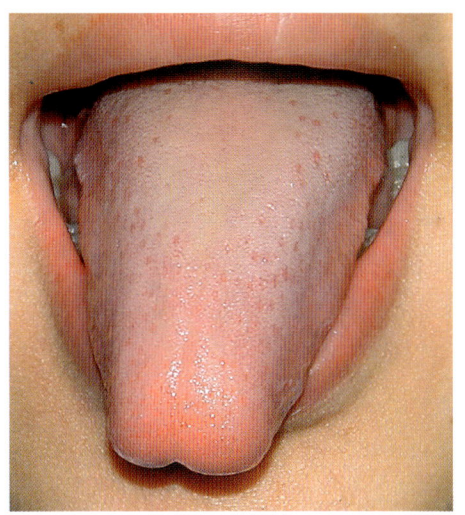

图(See color fig)2.3.4.3   图(See color fig)2.3.4.4

5. 点、刺舌
5. The Spotted or Prickled Tongue

点，是指蕈状乳头增大，数目增多，乳头充血水肿，大者称星，称红星舌(图 2.3.5.1)；小者称点，称红点舌(图 2.3.5.2)；刺，是指蕈状乳头增大、高突，并形成尖锋，形如芒刺，摸之棘手，称为芒刺舌(图 2.3.5.3)。点和刺相似，时常并见，合称点刺舌。多因邪热亢盛、脏腑热极、瘟毒入血、湿热蕴于血分所致。一般点刺愈多，邪热愈甚。

Red spot tongue also named red star tongue, is called because of enlarged, numerous and congested mushroom papilla on the surface of the tongue, the big one is named as star (See color fig. 2.3.5.1) while the small spot (See color fig. 2.3.5.2). The hyperplasic lingual papillae, protruding like the thorns and causing a prickly sensation when they are palpated with finger are known as the prickled tongue (See color fig. 2.3.5.3). Because they are similar and can be seen at the same time, so they are usually called as spotted and prickled tongue. They

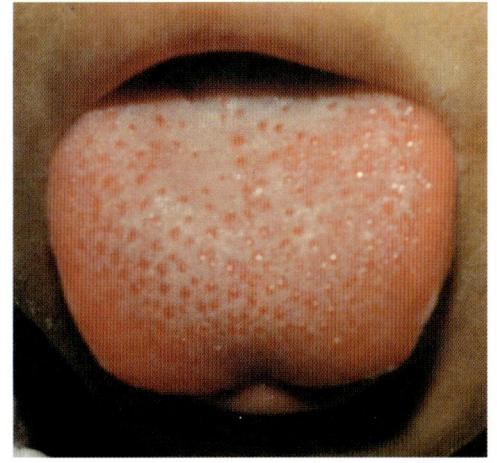

图(See color fig)2.3.5.1

are mostly caused by excessive heat evils, or extreme heat in *Zang-Fu*, or the attack into the blood by pestilence poisoning or stagnation of damp-heat in blood. The more exorbitant the heat evils are, the more and larger the awn-prickles are.

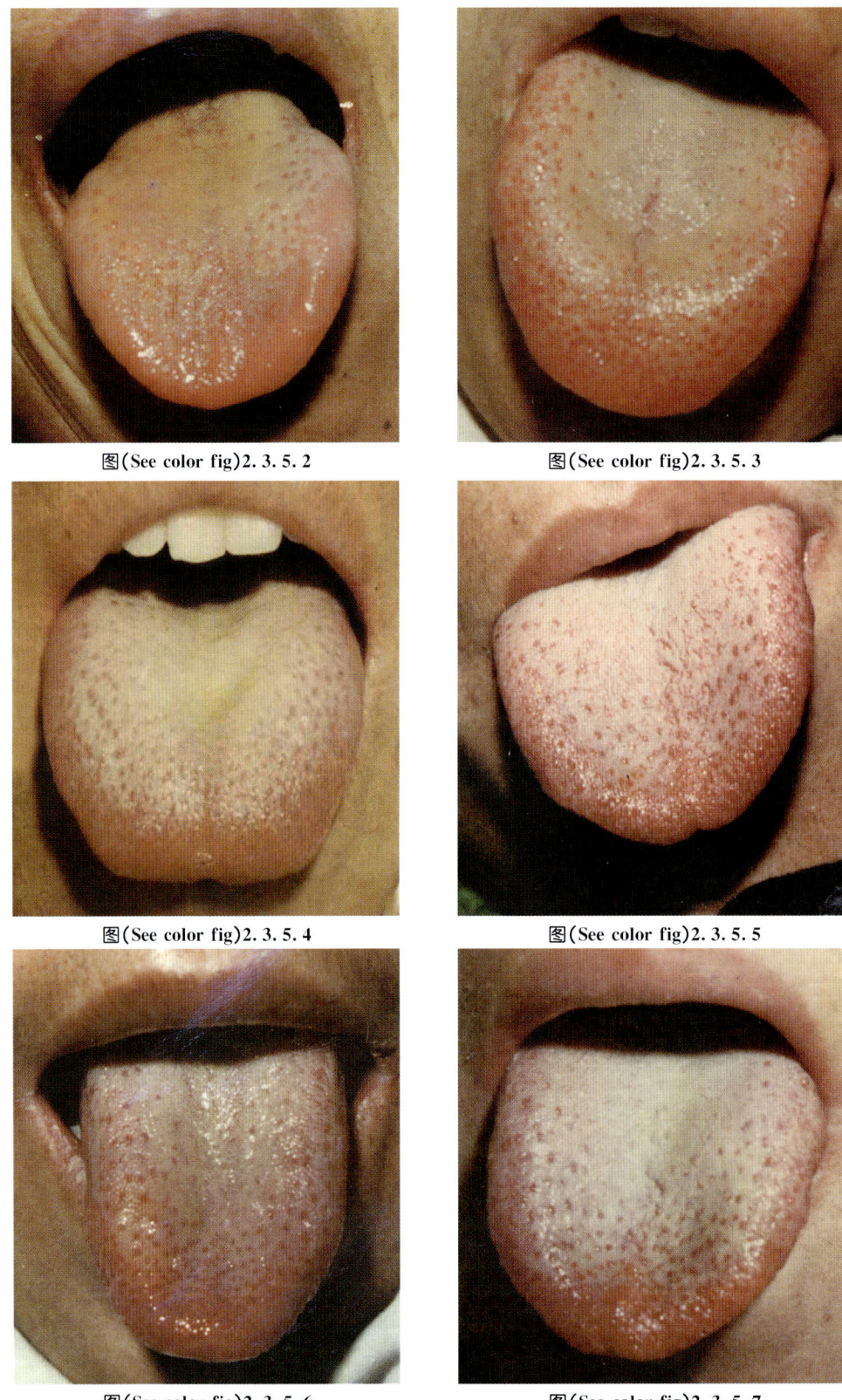

图(See color fig)2.3.5.2

图(See color fig)2.3.5.3

图(See color fig)2.3.5.4

图(See color fig)2.3.5.5

图(See color fig)2.3.5.6

图(See color fig)2.3.5.7

舌红而点刺散在,为气分热极(图 2.3.5.4);舌绛而红星或芒刺满布,为热入营血,气血壅滞(图 2.3.5.5);舌绛有黑点刺者,为热毒已极,将发斑疹之征象(图 2.3.5.6)。

A red tongue with scattered spots and prickles suggests excessive heat in the *qi* (See color fig. 2.3.5.4). A crimson tongue with prickles spreading the whole body means heat invasion into *yin* and blood and resulting in stagnation of *qi* and blood (See color fig. 2.3.5.5). A crimson tongue with dark prickles suggest the excessive heat evils and coming on maculae (See color fig. 2.3.5.6).

舌尖有点刺,多为心火亢盛(图 2.3.5.7);舌边有点刺,多为肝胆火旺(图 2.3.5.8);多中有点刺,为胃肠热盛(图 2.3.5.9)。

Prickles on tongue tip are due to flaring fire in the heart (See color fig. 2.3.5.7). Prickles on the sides of tongue are due to heat in the liver and gallbladder (See color fig. 2.3.5.8). Prickles on middle tongue are due to heat in the stomach and intestines (See color fig. 2.3.5.9).

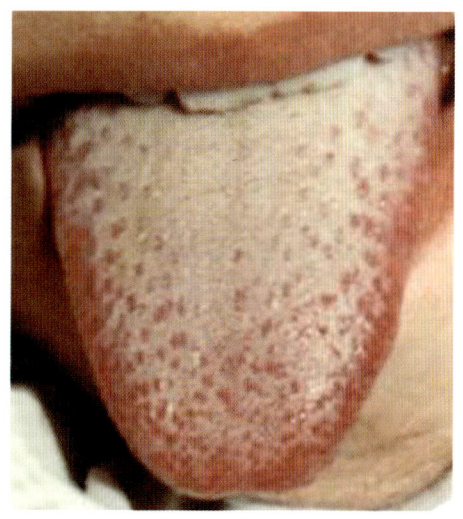

图(See color fig)2.3.5.8

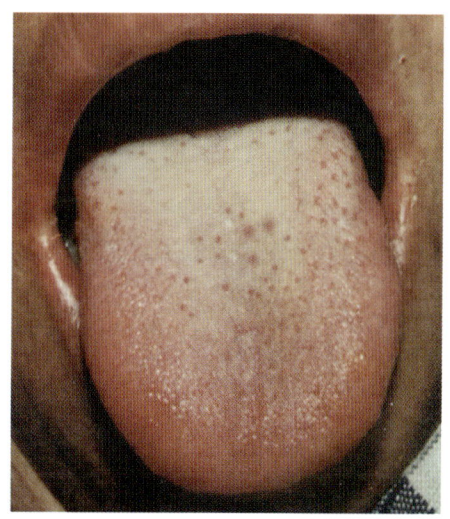

图(See color fig)2.3.5.9

6. 裂纹舌
6. The Fissured Tongue

舌面上呈现多少不等,深浅不一,形状各异的裂沟或皱纹,沟裂中无舌苔覆盖,称为裂纹舌(图 2.3.6.1)。多因血虚失养、热灼津伤和阴液亏虚所致。

If there are cracks in different size, depth and shape, on which without any fur cover, it is called a crack tongue (See color fig. 2.3.6.1). It is caused by deficient blood failing to manifest the tongue surface, or fluid injury and deficient blood *yin* resulting from excessive heat.

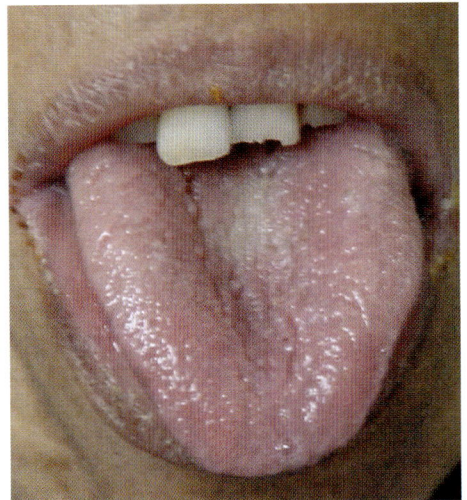

图(See color fig)2.3.6.1

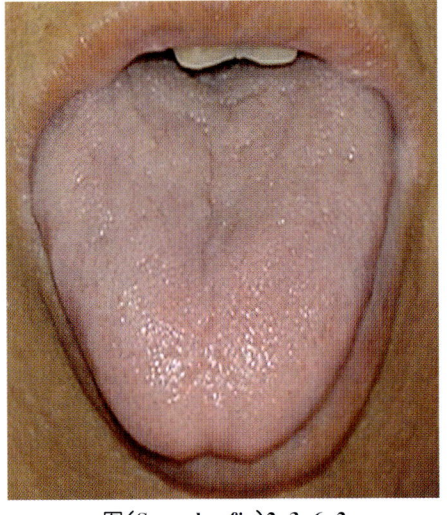

图(See color fig)2.3.6.2

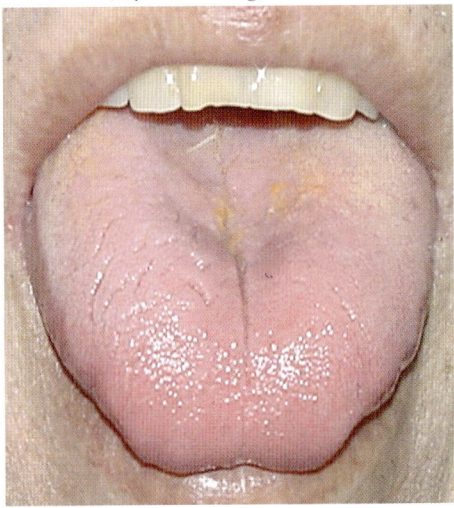

图(See color fig)2.3.6.3

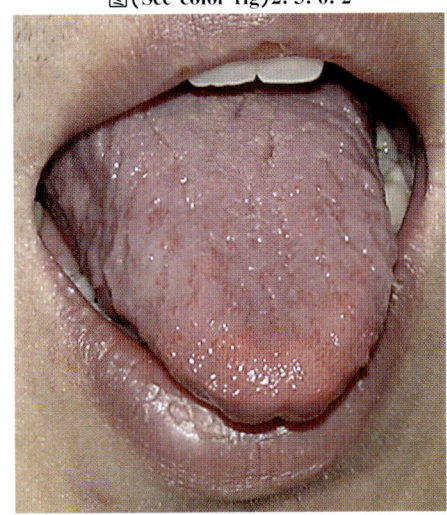

图(See color fig)2.3.6.4

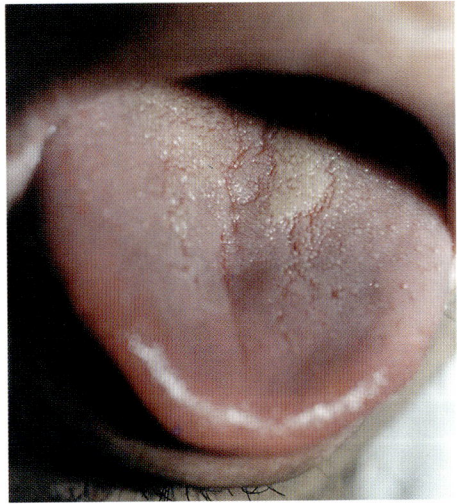

图(See color fig)2.3.6.5

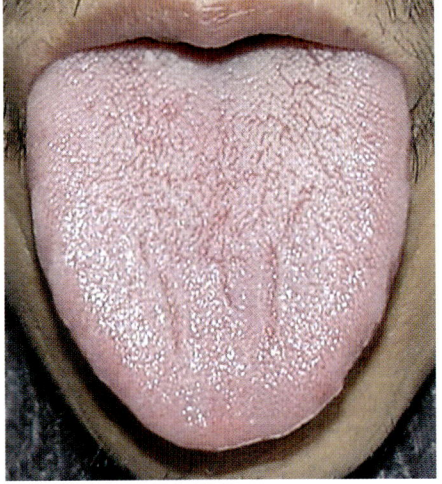

图(See color fig)2.3.6.6

舌色淡白而有裂纹或裂沟者,为血虚之候(图 2.3.6.2);若舌红赤而有裂纹或裂沟,舌面有黄厚苔者,为脏腑实热,热灼津伤(图 2.3.6.3);若舌绛无苔而舌面有裂纹或裂沟者,为阴虚液涸(图 2.3.6.4)、(图 2.3.6.5)。

The pale tongue with fissures suggests deficiency of blood (See color fig. 2.3.6.2). The dark red tongue with fissures and thick yellow fur on the surface means excess heat in *Zang-Fu* which consume the fluid (See color fig. 2.3.6.3). The crimson tongue with fissures on the surface but without any fur indicates exhaustion of *yin* fluid (See color fig. 2.3.6.4),(See color fig. 2.3.6.5).

若舌质淡红,而舌有较浅的裂纹,裂纹中一般有苔覆盖,且无不适感觉者,为先天性舌裂(图 2.3.6.6)。应与病理性裂纹相鉴别。

The pale red tongue with light cracks on the surface on which is covered with fur, and without any unsuitable syndromes are formed at birth (See color fig. 2.3.6.6). We should distinguish them from the pathological fissures by asking patients.

7. 齿痕舌
7. The Teeth Printed Tongue

舌体边缘有牙齿压迫的痕迹,称为齿痕舌或齿印舌(图 2.3.7.1)。多因脾虚、水湿内盛所致。

The tongue with tooth prints at its borders is known as teeth-printed tongue as a result of the pressure of dental coronae upon the puffy tongue (See color fig. 2.3.7.1). It mostly results from spleen deficiency and excessive dampness.

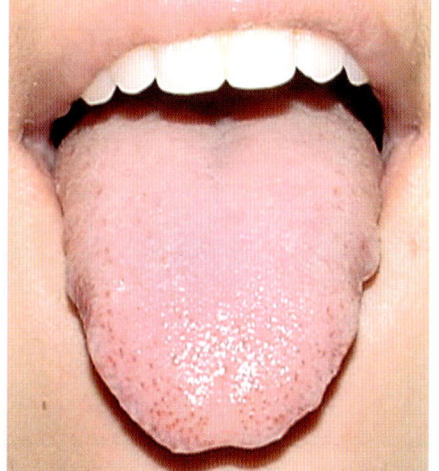

图(See color fig)2.3.7.1

齿痕舌多与胖大舌并见,若舌体淡而舌边有齿痕,多为寒湿内盛(图 2.3.7.2);若舌红而肿胀满口,舌边有齿痕,为内有湿热痰浊壅滞(图 2.3.7.3)。

Therefore, the teeth-printed tongue often coexists with the puffy one. The pale and moist tongue with tooth prints at its borders usually suggests an excess of cold of cold-dampness (See color fig. 2.3.7.2), whereas the red and enlarged tongue filling up the mouth with tooth marks on its margin, suggest the stagnation of internal damp-heat and phlegm (See color fig. 2.3.7.3).

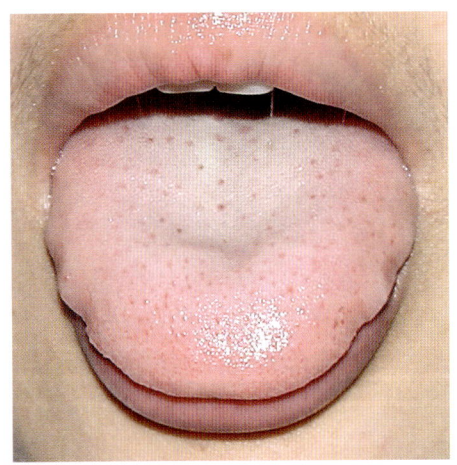
图(See color fig) 2.3.7.2

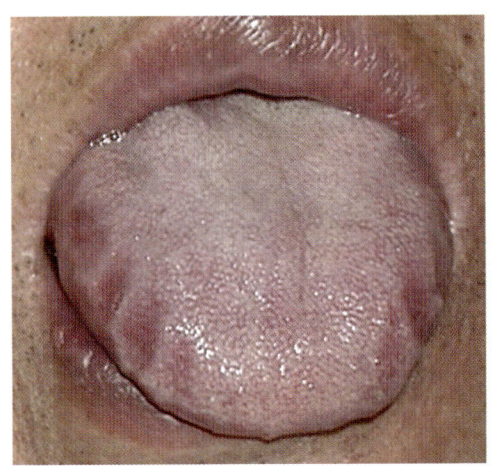
图(See color fig) 2.3.7.3

第四节 诊 舌 态
Section 4　Observation of The Moving State of The Tongue

舌态，即舌体运动时的状态。正常舌态特征为活动灵敏，伸缩自如，是气血充盛，经脉通调，脏腑健旺的表现。若出现舌体痿软、强硬、㖞斜、颤动、吐弄、短缩、弛纵等异常舌态，多为病态。

The state of the tongue is the tongue normal movement. The normal state of the tongue characterizes as stretching and shortening smoothly, which suggest sufficient *qi* and blood, smooth channels and vigorous *Zang-Fu*. The common abnormal changes of moving state are as follows: atrophy, stiffness, wryness, tremor, protruding and licking, shortness and so on, and suggest pathogenic states.

1. 痿软舌
1. The Flaccid Tongue

舌体软弱无力，不能随意伸缩回旋，称为痿软舌（图2.4.1.1）。多因气血两亏、热灼津伤、阴液亏虚，舌肌失养所致。《灵枢·经脉》指出："肌肉软，则舌痿"。

The weak tongue unable to protrude and curl is called flaccid tongue resulting mostly from the tongue body not being nourished due to protracted deficiency of *qi* and blood or consumption of *yin* fluid due to excessive heat (See color fig. 2.4.1.1). *The Chapter in Spirit Pirot says*: "Muscles atrophy result in weak and flaccid tongue."

舌体痿软舌色淡白者，为气血两虚，久病舌体失养（图2.4.1.2）；若舌体痿软而舌红苔黄者，是热灼津伤（图2.4.1.3）；即如《辨舌指南》所说："暴痿多由于热灼，故常出现红干之舌"。舌体痿软而舌绛光滑者，外感病属热极伤阴，内伤病属阴虚火旺（图2.4.1.4）。

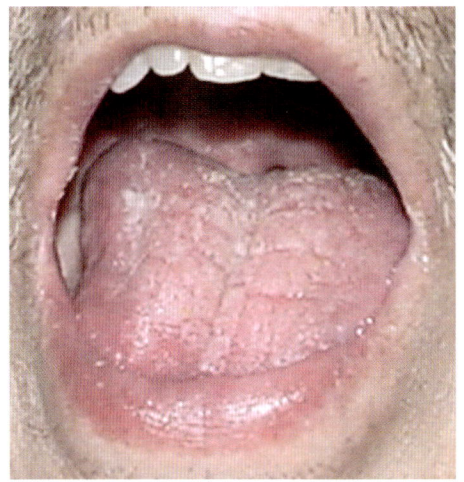 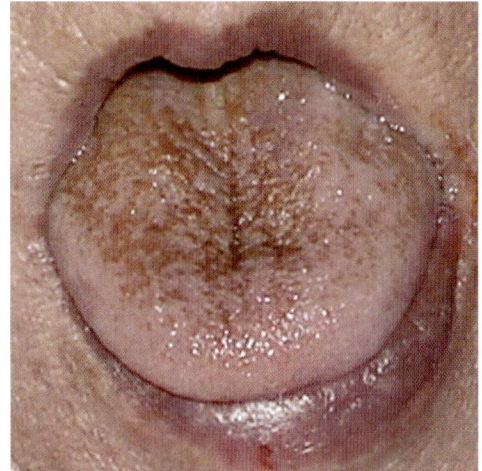

图(See color fig)2.4.1.1　　　　　　　　图(See color fig)2.4.1.2

The flaccid tongue with pale color in chronic diseases usually is due to deficiency of both *qi* and blood, because of malnutrition of muscles, tendons and vessels (See color fig. 2.4.1.2). The flaccid tongue in red color with yellow fur is due to injury of body fluid consumed by excessive heat (See color fig. 2.4.1.3). Just as *the guides for tongue diagnose* had said: "the abruptly dry and red-crimson tongue most probably indicates extremely intense pathogenic heat with impairment of *yin* fluid." The smooth and flaccid tongue in crimson color usually belongs to impairment of *yin* because of extremely intense pathogenic heat in exogenous diseases, but the flaring fire because of deficient *yin* in diseases due to internal injury (See color fig. 2.4.1.4).

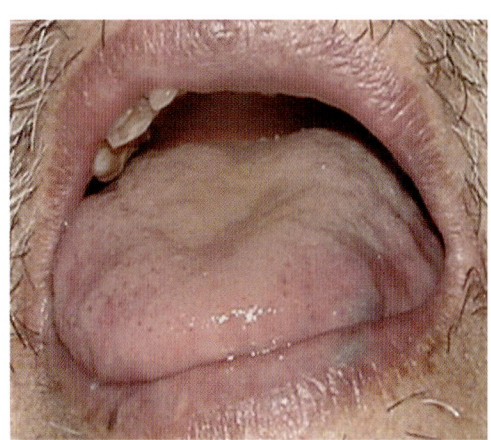 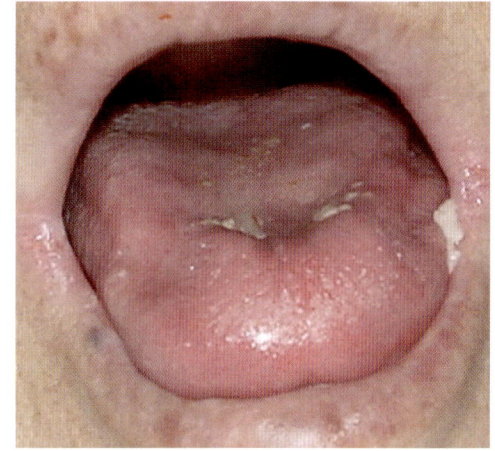

图(See color fig)2.4.1.3　　　　　　　　图(See color fig)2.4.1.4

2. 强硬舌
2. The Stiff Tongue

舌体失柔和,卷伸不利,或板硬强直,不能转动,称为强硬舌(图2.4.2.1)。多因热入心包、高热伤津、或风痰阻络所致。由于舌能调节发声,故强硬舌常与语言謇涩并见。

It is an inflexible tongue with difficulty in moving or inability of turning. As the tongue participates in the articulation of voice, the patient with stiff tongue frequently suffers from slurred speech (See color fig. 2.4.2.1). It mostly results from an attack of the pericardium by excessive heat, heat impairment of body fluid because of extremely intense pathogenic heat, or wind-phlegm obstructing the meridians in tongue.

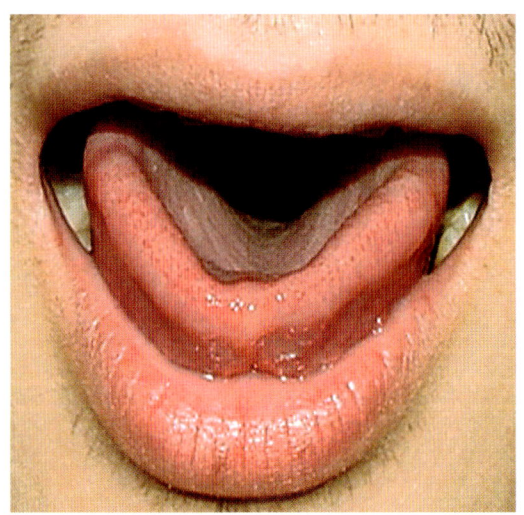

图(See color fig)2.4.2.1

舌体强硬而舌质深红,伴有高热者,为热入心包,或高热伤津(图2.4.2.2);舌体强硬伴有舌胖苔厚腻者,为痰浊内阻(图2.4.2.3)。

The stiff tongue in dark red color with high fever is due to the attack of the pericardium by excessive heat or the impairment body fluid by extremely intense pathogenic heat (See color fig. 2.4.2.2). The enlarged and stiff tongue with yellow greasy coating always results from phlegm obstructing the meridians (See color fig. 2.4.2.3).

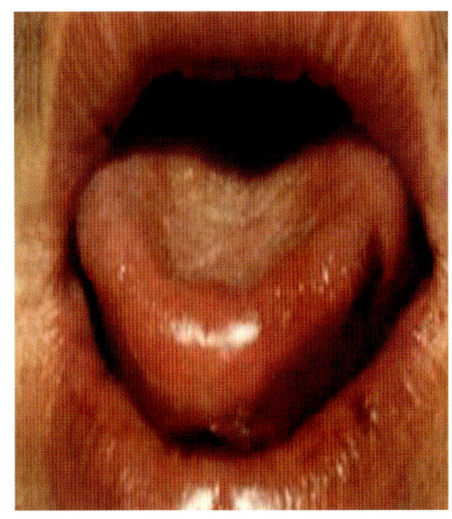 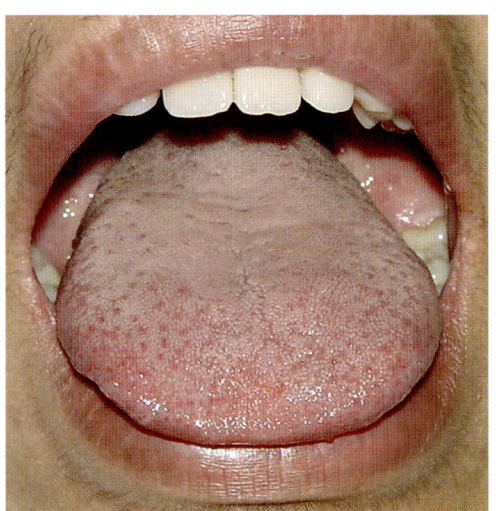

图(See color fig)2.4.2.2　　　　图(See color fig.)2.4.2.3

《千金方》说:"舌强不能言,病在脏腑"。《辨舌指南》指出:"凡红舌强硬,为脏腑实热已极。"

A Thousand Gold Worthy had said: "A patient can't speak with stiff tongue this diseases lie in Zang-Fu." And The guides for Tongue Diagnosis had referred: "all the stiff tongue red color is due to extreme excessive heat in *Zang-Fu*."

3. 歪斜舌
3. The Wry Tongue

伸舌时舌体歪向一侧,称为歪斜舌。多因肝风内动,夹痰夹瘀,痰瘀阻滞一侧经络所致。由于痰瘀阻滞的一侧舌肌弛缓,无力收缩,而健侧舌肌如常,故伸舌时向健侧歪斜。多见于中风或中风先兆。常与口眼㖞斜,肢体偏瘫同时出现。

A tongue turning to one side involuntarily while protruding is called the wry tongue (See color fig. 2.4.3.1), in most cases with marked inclination of the anterior half the tongue to either the left or the right side. This morbid tongue is mostly caused by obstruction of the collaterals on one side of the tongue body due to the liver-wind stirring up inside the body with upward stagnation of phlegm of blood stasis. Since the muscles on the affected side of the tongue are sluggish and weak and turns to the healthy side while protruding. It often indicates apoplexy or a premonitory sign of apoplexy, and it often comes in to being with wry mouth, distorted eyes and hemiplegia at the same time.

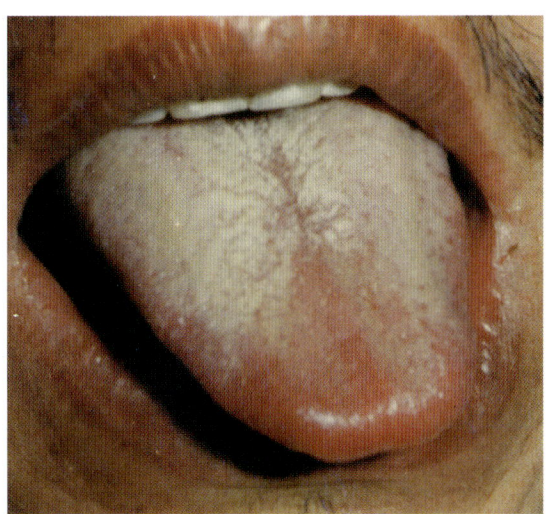

图(See color fig)2.4.3.1

舌体偏歪,舌质紫红,来势急骤者,为肝风发痉(图2.4.3.1);舌体偏歪,舌质淡红,来势缓慢者,为中风偏枯(图2.4.3.2);单见舌体歪斜,多是中风先兆(图2.4.3.3)。

If it occurs suddenly and the tongue is red or purple, it is a condition of convulsion due to liver wind (See color fig. 2.4.3.1). While it occurs gradually and the tongue is pale, it is a condition of hemiplegia of wind-stroke (See color fig. 2.4.3.2). The tongue is only wry mostly due to sign of wind-stroke (See color fig. 2.4.3.3).

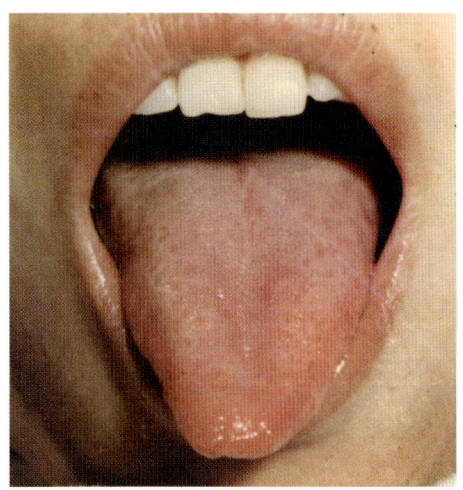 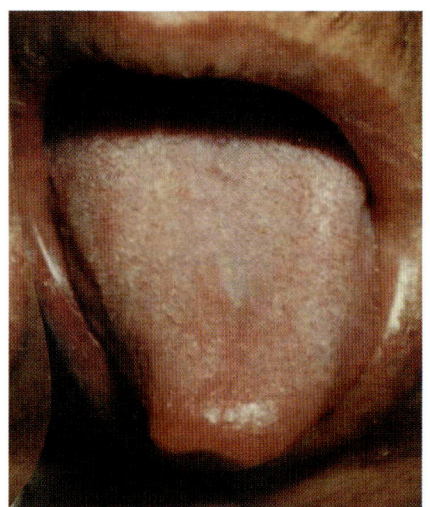

图(See color fig)2.4.3.2　　　　　　　图(See color fig)2.4.3.3

《辨舌指南》指出："若舌紫红势急者,由肝风发痉,宜熄风镇痉,色淡红势缓者,由中风偏枯;若舌偏歪语塞,口眼㖞斜,半身不遂者,偏风也。"

The Guide for Tongue Diagnosis had said, "It occurs suddenly and the tongue is red or purple, it is a condition of convulsion due to liver wind and drugs with the function of calming the liver wind should be used. While it occurs gradually and the tongue is pale, it is a condition of hemiplegia or wind-stroke. The wry tongue comes into being with the syndromes of wry mouth, distorted eyes and hemiplegia suggest wind-stroke."

4. 颤动舌
4. The Trembling Tongue

舌体震颤抖动,不能自主,称为颤动舌。轻者仅伸舌时颤动;重者不伸舌时亦抖颤难以自主。多因血虚、阴亏、阳亢、热盛等致舌体失养、风阳内动所致。多为肝风内动的征象。

It refers to shivering in light diseases and even swaying that are not controlled by the patient in serious diseases. It is also called "tremor". It mostly results from deficient blood and *yin* due to malnutrition of the tongue body, or liver wind and yang stirring internally caused by excessive heat and ascending hyperactivity of *yang*. It is always a sign of liver wind stirring internally.

舌淡白而颤动者,多属血虚动风;舌红少津而颤动者,多属阴虚动风、肝阳化风。舌绛而颤动者,多属热极生风,另外,酒毒内蕴,亦可见舌体颤动。

The trembling tongue in pale color is due to internal wind caused by deficient blood, while the trembling tongue in red color with little fluid on the suffers is often due to internal wind cause by deficient yin or the transformation from *liver-yang*.

Tremor in red or crimson tongue is often due to extreme heat which damages the body-fluid and leads to internal wind stirring. It is also seen in alcohol intoxication.

5. 吐弄舌
5. The Protruding And Licking Tongue

舌伸于口外，不即回缩者，称为吐舌（图2.4.5.1）；舌反复吐而即回，或舌舐口唇四周，掉动不宁者，称为弄舌（图2.4.5.2）。多因心脾有热，灼伤津液，肝筋失养，引动肝风，致筋脉动摇而不能自主。或津伤精亏，舌体失养，舌体紧涩，患者每欲吐弄以舒缓之。

The tongue which stretches out of mouth and can't retracts into mouth immediately is called a protruding tongue (See color fig. 2.4.5.1). The tongue that stretches out and immediately retracts into mouth or licks the lips and corners of the mouth is called a lick tongue (See color fig. 2.4.5.2). It usually results from excess heat in heart and spleen consumption the body fluid, which fails to nourish the liver tendons and leads to internal liver wind stirring or impairment of body fluid and consumption of essence failing to nourish the tongue body and leading to the tongue contracting. So the patients have to protrude or lick one's tongue to extend it.

吐舌不宁，多属疫毒攻心，或正气已绝；弄舌不已，多见于小儿智力发育不全。或为动风之先兆。

The frequent protrusion of the tongue is usually seen in cases of attack of the heart by the pestilential heat or exhaustion of the vital *qi* (See color fig. 2.4.5.2), and playing with the tongue is considered as a sign of wind-stroke or in infants with poor mental development.

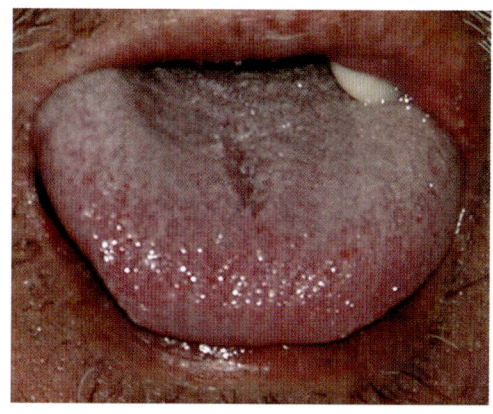

图(See color fig)2.4.5.1

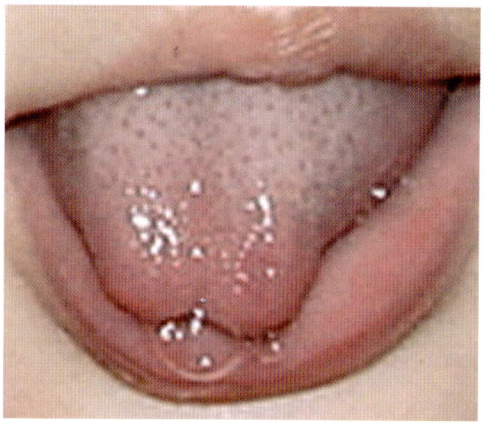

图(See color fig)2.4.5.2

6. 短缩舌
6. The Shortened Tongue

舌体紧缩不能伸长,甚则舌体抵齿都很困难,称为短缩舌(图2.4.6.1)。多因寒凝筋脉、气血亏虚或热盛伤津,筋脉挛急所致。常与痿软舌并见。

The tongue which contracts and shortens, and is unable to stretch, even can't reach teeth is called a shortened tongue (See color fig. 2.4.6.1). It is usually caused by cold coagulating in meridians and contracture of tendons, resulting from deficient *qi* and blood, or excessive heat impairing the body fluid. It usually can be seen with the flaccid tongue at the same time.

图(See color fig)2.4.6.1

舌体短缩,舌色淡白或青紫而湿润,为寒凝筋脉,舌脉挛缩(图2.4.6.1);舌体短缩,舌色淡白胖嫩者,为脾虚不运,气血亏虚,筋脉失养(图2.4.6.2);舌体短缩,舌红或绛而干燥者,为热盛伤津,筋脉挛急(图2.4.6.3)。

The shortened moist tongue in pale or bluish purple color is due to cold coagulated in meridians and contracture of the tongue tendons (See color fig. 2.4.6.1). The shortened, fat and tender tongue in pale color is due to deficiency of *qi* and blood or insufficient spleen failing to nourish the tongue tendons (See color fig. 2.4.6.2). The shortened and dry tongue in red or crimson color is due to body fluid impairment by excessive heat causing the contracture of the tendons and meridians (See color fig. 2.4.6.3).

此外,先天性舌系带过短,亦可出现舌卷不伸,称为绊舌,无辨证意义。应与短缩舌相鉴别。《辨舌指南》说:"凡舌短由于生就者,无关寿夭。"因病短缩,则多属危候。

Besides, shortened frenulum linguae congenitally all leads to the tongue curling, which is harmless and should be distinguished from the shorten tongue. *The Guides for the Tongue Diagnosis* had said:"If the shortened tongue is inborn, it has no connection with the short life." If it occurs in diseases, no matter what condition it is, it's a critical case.

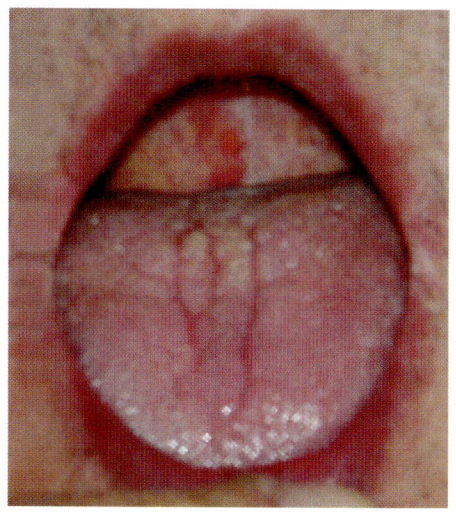
图(See color fig)2.4.6.2

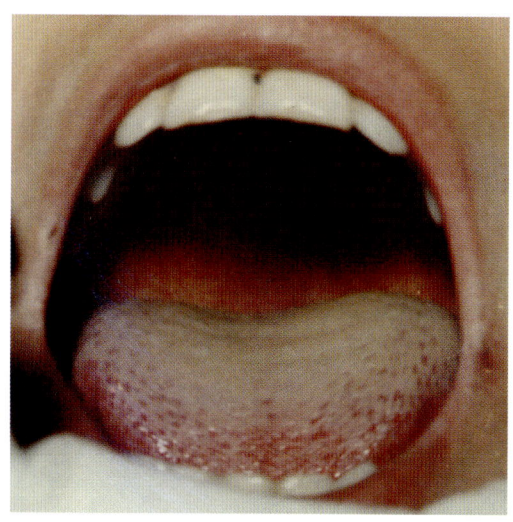
图(See color fig)2.4.6.3

第五节　诊舌下络脉
Section 5　Observations of The Vessels Below Tongue

舌下络脉,指舌下位于舌系带两侧纵行的大络脉。正常人舌下络脉仅隐现于舌下,管径小于27mm,其长度亦不超过舌尖至舌下肉阜的五分之三,其颜色为淡紫色,脉络无怒张、紧束、弯曲、增生,排列有序。绝大多数为单支,极少有双支出现(图2.5.1.1)。

Hypoglossal vessels are referred as the two thick bluish purple vessels that can be seen beside the frenulum of tongue in normal condition. Their diameter is no more than 27millimeter. Their length is no more than three fifth of the length from tongue tip to sublingual caruncle. Their color is pale purple and

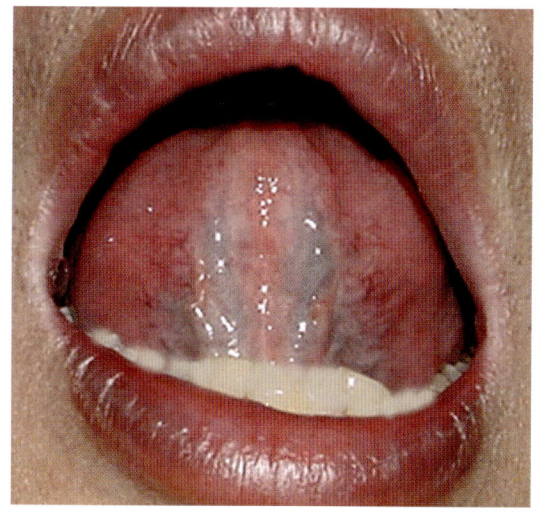
图(See color fig)2.5.1.1

there is no varicosity, contracture, curve, hyperplasia and disorder in range. Most of them are single branch and little of them two branches (See color fig. 2.5.1.1).

诊舌下络脉主要观察其长度、形态、色泽、粗细、舌下小血络等变化,以帮助诊断疾病。

The observation of the hypoglossal vessels means observing changes of the length, state, color, thickness and small vessels below the tongue, in order to help the clinical doctors to diagnose diseases.

1. 舌下络脉的观察方法
1. Methods of Observing The Vessels Below Tongue

令病人张开口,舌体向上腭方向翘起,舌尖轻抵上腭或门齿内侧,勿用力太过,使舌体保持自然放松,舌下络脉充分显露(图2.5.1.2)。仔细察看舌下络脉的长短、粗细、形态、颜色等变化,有无怒张、弯曲等异常改变,周围细小络脉的颜色、形态有无异常。

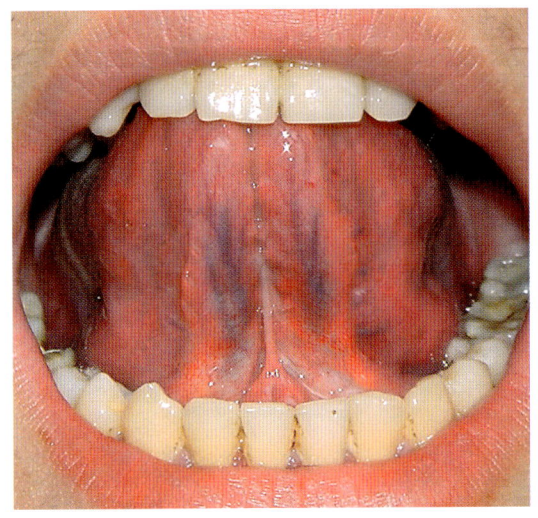

图(See color fig)2.5.1.2

Patients should open their mouth, raise their tongue body upward to palate, and reach the tongue tip to the upper palate or the inside of the front teeth softly, keep the tongue body relaxed and expose the vessels below the tongue sufficiently (See color fig. 2.5.1.2). The inspector should observe not only changes of length, thickness, state, size and color of vessels below the tongue and the small vessels nearby, but also the abnormality of varicosity and curve.

2. 舌下络脉异常及其临床意义
2. The Clinical Significance of Abnormal Hypoglossal Vessels

舌下络脉短而细,周围小络脉不明显,舌色偏淡者,多属气血不足,脉络不充(图2.5.2.1);下络脉粗胀,呈青紫、绛、绛紫、紫黑色,舌下细小络脉呈暗红色或紫色网络,舌下络脉曲张如紫色珠子状大小不等的结节等改变,皆为血瘀的征象(图2.5.2.2)、(图2.5.2.3);多因气滞、寒凝、热郁、痰湿、气虚、阳虚等所致,需结合其他症状综合分析。

The pale tongue with the shortened and thin hypoglossal vessels, and there being no vessels nearby mostly suggest insufficient *qi* and blood failing to full the vessels (See color fig. 2.5.2.1). If the vessels become thicker and their color become bluish purple, crimson,

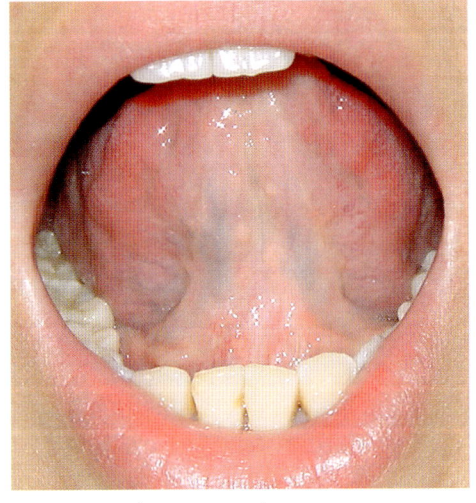

图(See color fig)2.5.2.1

crimson to purple, or dark purple, or there are dark red or purple netted small vessels below the tongue, or there are changes of tubercle like purple pearls in inequality of size of hypoglossal vessels, it is sign of blood stasis (See color fig. 2.5.2.2) (See color fig. 2.5.2.3). Which is due to the stagnation of *qi*, accumulation of cold, phlegm and heat, or the deficiency of *qi* and *yang*. The doctors should analyze these changes combining with other clinical syndromes.

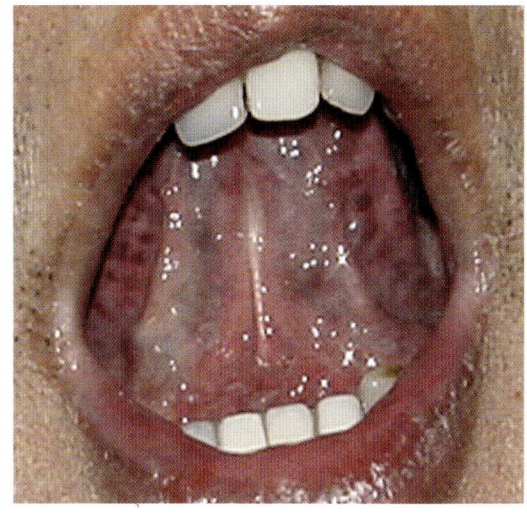
图(See color fig)2.5.2.2

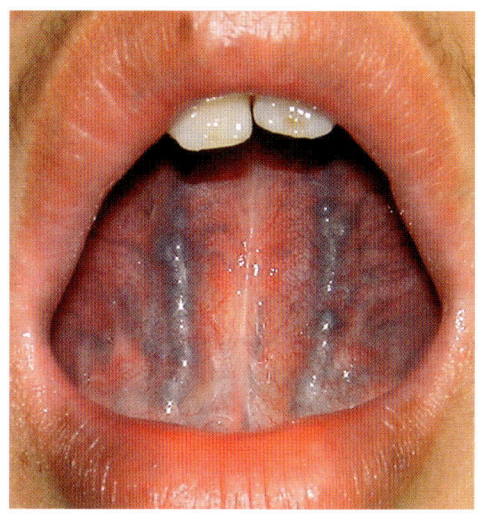
图(See color fig)2.5.2.3

舌下络脉的变化，有时会早于舌色变化，因此，舌下络脉是分析气血运行情况的重要依据，对血虚、瘀血等的辨证有较大的意义。

The changes of hypoglossal come into being early than the tongue's colors. So observation of the hypoglossal vessels is an important basis to analyze the movement of *qi* and blood, and it is significant to the differentiation of insufficient blood and blood stasis.

第三章 诊 舌 苔

Chapter 3 Observations of The Tongue Coating

舌苔,指舌面上附着的一层苔状物。正常舌苔是由脾胃之生气上熏,胃津上潮,凝聚于舌面所生。如章虚谷在《伤寒论本旨·辨舌苔》中说:"舌苔由胃中生气所致,而胃气由心脾发生,故无病之人常有薄苔,是胃中之生气,如地上之微草也。"病理舌苔也与胃气之上升有关,但往往因病变而夹有食浊之气,诸病邪气上泛而成。故章虚谷又说:"胃有生气,而邪入之,则苔即长厚,如草根之得秽浊而长发也。"

The tongue coating is a layer of fur-like substance covering the surface by the *spleen-qi* and *stomach-qi*, and the coagulating action of the stomach-fluid on the tongue surface. As *Zhang Xugu*, who had written the book *Original meaning of Cold-Attack · the Differentiation of the Tongue Coating* said, "Tongue coating is made up of *stomach-qi* which rise from heart and spleen. So normal person always has thin fur. It means the *stomach-qi* is vigorous. It is just like grass growing in fertile soil." The abnormal coating is also formed from the ascending *stomach-qi*, but which is made up of *stomach-qi* and steaming up evils in combination. Just as *Zhang Xugu* has said: "The coating becomes thicker because of *stomach-qi* and steaming up evils in combination. It is just like the grass root that grows vigorously in dirty and turbid soil."

人以胃气为本,胃为水谷之海,五脏六腑之气皆受气于胃,胃气之变可以影响全身脏腑、气血、经络。而苔又是胃气熏蒸所化,故脏腑病变均能反映于舌苔之上。即如《形色外诊简摩》所说:"苔乃胃气之所熏蒸,五脏皆禀气于胃,故可借以诊五脏之寒热虚实也。"通过诊舌苔变化,可以推测病邪的性质,病位的浅深,津液的盈亏,邪气的消长,病情的进退,预后的善恶,为诊治疾病提供依据。

A human body's essence is the *qi* of the stomach, and stomach is always called as "the reservoir of water and food". *Qi* of *Five-Zang* and *Six-Fu* all comes from stomach. The changes of stomach-qi can influence on the *Zang-Fu*, *qi* and blood, channels. The coating is formed under the steaming action of the stomach *qi*. So the changes of tongue coating may inflect the diseases of *the Five Zang-Viscera* and *Six-Fu Viscera*. Just as *Simple Estimate on Exterior Diagnosis of Shape and Color* has said, "the coating is formed under the steaming action of the stomach-*qi*. *Qi* of *the Five Zang-Viscera* and *Six-Fu Viscera* all arise from stomach. So we can diagnose the cold, heat, insufficiency of excess of the *Five Zang-Viscera*." The significances of observing the coating are as follows: to predict the character of the evil, to detect the location of the disease, to infer the tendency of disease, to judge the sufficiency or insufficiency of the body fluid, to distinguish the exuberance or decline of the evil, to know the coating can provide significant basis to diagnose diseases.

正常的舌苔，一般是薄白均匀，干湿适中，舌面的中部和根部稍厚。由于患者的胃气有强弱，病邪有寒热，故可形成各种不同的病理性舌苔。

A normal fur, white in color and even in distribution is spread thinly on the surface of the tongue, not too wet and not spread thinly on the surface of the tongue, not too wet and not too dry, a little thick on the middle and root of the tongue various morbid tongue fur can be formed because of the patient's vigorous or weak *stomach-qi* and the cold or heat evils.

诊舌苔，以望诊为主，必要时可采用扪摸揩刮等方法以辅助诊断。要注意苔质和苔色两方面的变化。

Observation is the major method to inspect the coating touching, scraping methods should be used at necessary time observing tongue coating includes observing the color and the texture of coating.

第一节 诊 苔 质
Section 1 Observations of The Texture of Tongue Coating

苔质，是指舌苔的质地，形态。临床常见的苔质有厚薄、润燥、腻腐、剥落、真假等方面改变。

Observing coating texture is to observe the changes of vitality and shape of the coating. The changes includes the thick or thin, moist or dry, putrid or greasy, exfoliation, and true or false in clinic.

1. 薄苔、厚苔
1. Thickness and Thinness

舌苔的厚薄以"见底"、"不见底"作为衡量标准。透过舌苔能隐隐见到舌质者，称为薄苔（图 3.1.1.1）；不能透过舌苔见到舌质者，称为厚苔（图 3.1.1.2）。舌苔的厚薄，主要反映邪正的盛衰和邪气之深浅。

The "bottom can be seen" or "bottom can not be seen" is taken as the standard of judging thickness and thinness. The thin coating refers to that we can see the tongue body (bottom) indistinctly through the coating (See color fig. 3.1.1.1). The thick coating is a coating through which we cannot see the tongue body (See color fig. 3.1.1.2). Observing the thickness and thinness of coating is helpful to know the deep and shallow, the wax and wane of disease.

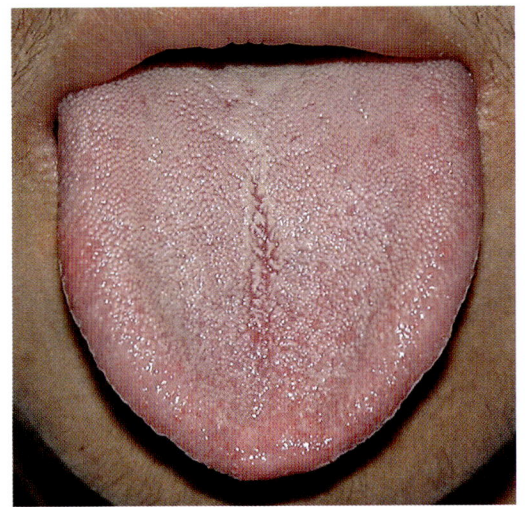

图(See color fig)3.1.1.1

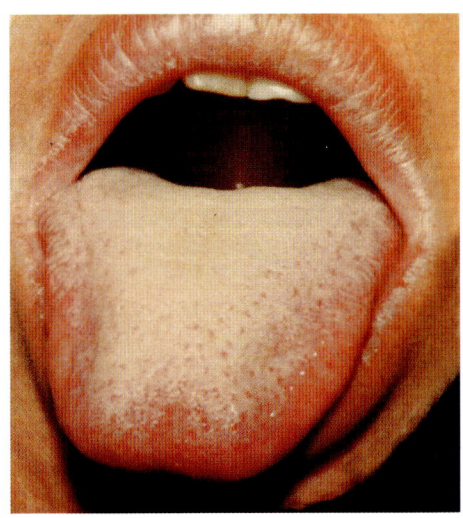

图(See color fig)3.1.1.2

舌苔薄而均匀,或中部稍厚,干湿适中,为正常人之舌苔的表现之一(图3.1.1.3),是胃气充盛、胃有生发之气的表现。

The thin and even fur, which is not too dry and not too wet, or a little thick in the middle of the tongue, is a sign of a healthy person (See color fig. 3.1.1.3). It suggests vigorous *stomach-qi* and active force in stomach.

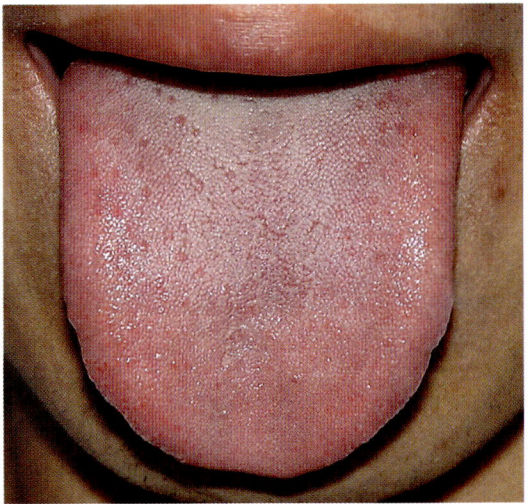

图(See color fig)3.1.1.3

舌苔厚是由胃气夹湿浊、痰浊、食浊、热邪等熏蒸,积滞舌面所致,多见于痰湿、食积、里热等证(图3.1.1.4)。《辨舌指南》说:"苔垢厚者,病气有余。"苔厚多为病邪入里,尤其是胃肠有积滞,苔厚更为明显(图3.1.1.5)。

The thick fur is formed by upward retention of dampness, phlegm, food and heat evils on the surface of the tongue due to rising up of the *stomach-qi*. It usually can be seen in the syndromes of phlegm-dampness, retention of food and interior heat etc (See color fig. 3.1.1.4). *The Guides for the Tongue Diagnosis* had said: "the thick and dirty fur means rich pathogenic factors." In most case, the thick fur suggests an interior syndrome. The thick fur will become more evident when there is retention in the gastrointestinal tract (See color fig. 3.1.1.5)

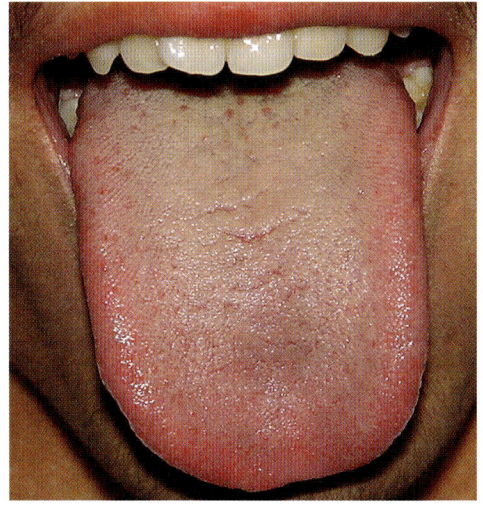

图(See color fig)3.1.1.4

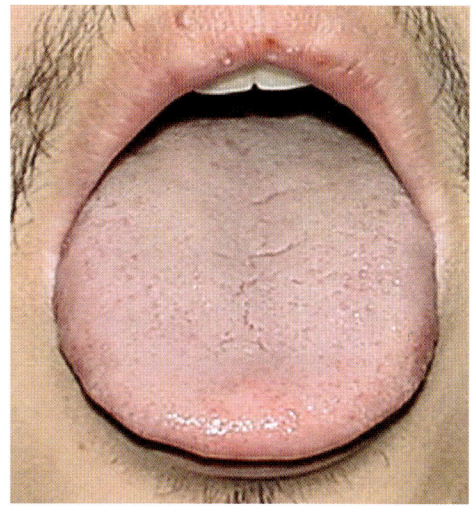

图(See color fig)3.1.1.5

辨舌苔厚薄可测邪气的深浅,苔薄在外感病中多属表证;在内伤病中多为病情轻浅,胃气未伤(图3.1.1.6);舌苔厚或舌中根部尤为显著者,多提示外感病邪气已入里,或胃肠内有宿食,或痰浊停滞(图3.1.1.7)。

Observing the thickness and thinness of coating is helpful to predict the deep and shallow of the evils. Generally speaking, when disease is in the exterior, or symptoms are mild and if the *stomach-qi* is not injured in the interior diseases the coating is often thin (See color fig. 3.1.1.6). Namely, thin coating suggests the exogenous exterior syndrome and mild syndrome of internal disease. When evils enter the interior, or there are retentions of phlegm or food in the gastrointestinal, the coating is usually especially found on the surface of the middle and root of the tongue (See color fig. 3.1.1.7).

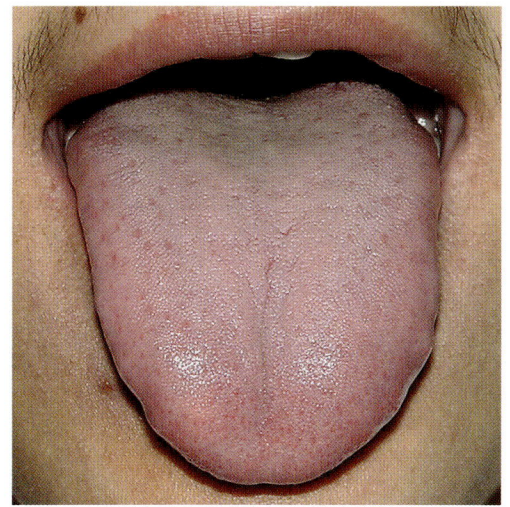

图(See color fig) 3.1.1.6

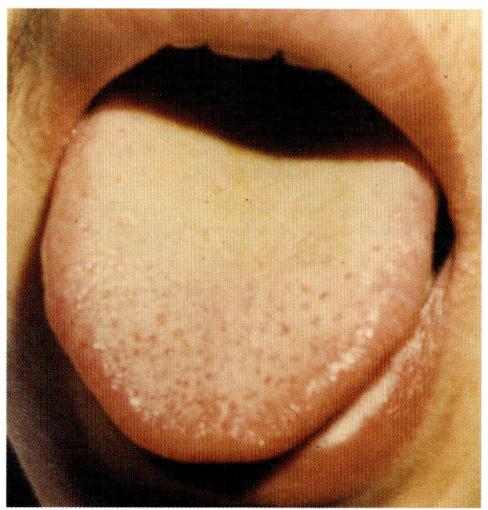

图(See color fig)3.1.1.7

辨舌苔厚薄的转化可辨病邪的进退,舌苔由薄转厚,提示邪气渐盛,或表邪入里,为病进或潜伏之邪开始暴露(图3.1.1.8)、(图3.1.1.9);舌苔由厚转薄,或舌上复生薄白新苔,提示正气胜邪,或里蕴之邪逐渐消退,为病退的征象(图3.1.1.10)、(图3.1.1.11)。

Observing the transformation of thickness and thinness of coating is helpful to distinguish the wax and wane of the evils. If thin coating becomes thick, it indicates that more vigorous evil enters the interior from the exterior and the disease changes from mild to severe, or the hidden evil becomes exposed and the disease is deteriorating (See color fig. 3.1.1.8) (See color fig. 3.1.1.9). While thick coating turns into thinor new thin white fur comes into being, it is a mark of evils being defeated by *vital-qi*, or evils being cleared up and the disease is improving (See color fig. 3.1.1.10) (See color fig. 3.1.1.11).

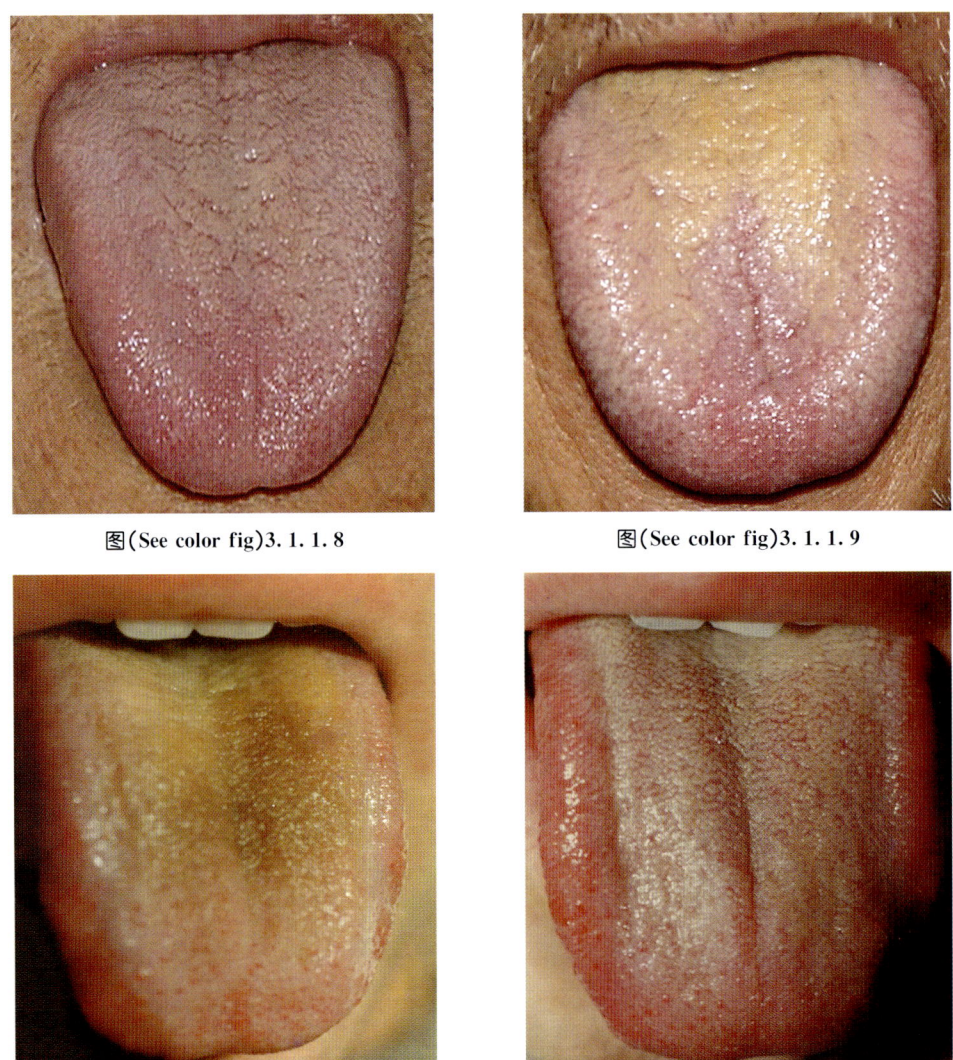

图(See color fig)3.1.1.8　　　　　　图(See color fig)3.1.1.9

图(See color fig)3.1.1.10　　　　　　图(See color fig)3.1.1.11

舌苔的厚薄转化,一般是渐变的过程,如薄苔突然增厚,提示邪气极盛,迅速入里(图3.1.1.12)、(图3.1.1.13);苔骤然消退,舌上无新生舌苔,为正不胜邪,或胃气暴绝(图

3.1.1.14)、(图 3.1.1.15)。

The transformation of thickness and thinness of coating is a slow changing course. If the thin fur gets thicker and thicker suddenly, it indicates extremely excessive evils enter the interior quickly (See color fig. 3.1.1.12) (See color fig. 3.1.1.13). If the fur is cleared up abruptly and new fur doesn't come into being, it indicates evils not being defeated by *vital-qi* or the sudden exhaustion of the *stomach-qi* (See color fig. 3.1.1.14) (See color fig. 3.1.1.15).

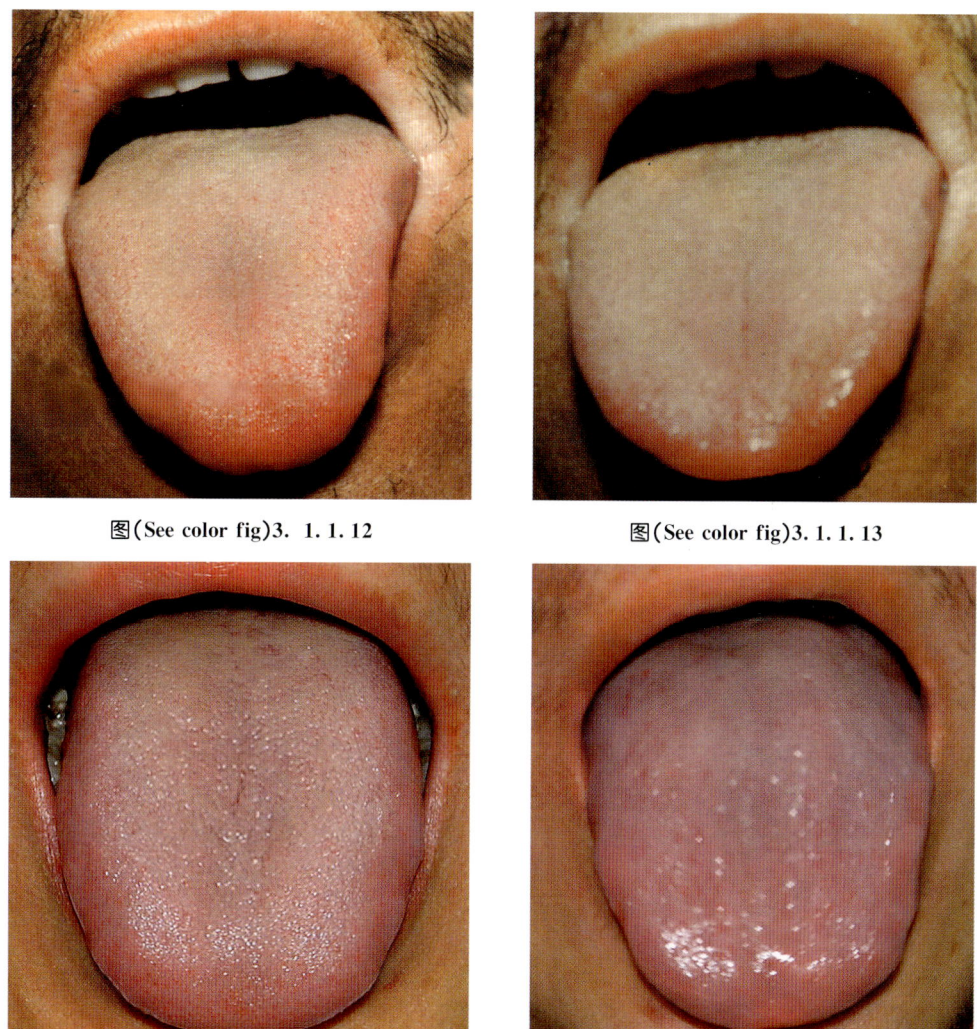

图(See color fig)3.1.1.12

图(See color fig)3.1.1.13

图(See color fig)3.1.1.14

图(See color fig)3.1.1.15

2. 润苔、燥苔
2. Moistness and Dryness

舌苔润泽有津,干湿适中,不滑不燥,称为润苔(图 3.1.2.1);舌面水分过多,伸舌欲滴,扪之湿滑,称为滑苔(图 3.1.2.2);舌苔干燥,扪之无津,甚则舌苔干裂,称为燥苔(图 3.1.2.3);苔质粗糙,扪之碍手,称为糙苔(图 3.1.2.4)。舌苔的润燥,主要反映体内津液的盈亏和输布情况。

The moistness and dryness reflect the wax and wane and the distribution of *body fluid*. The moist coating with moderate fluid on it, which is neither glossy nor dry, is named the moist fur (See color fig. 3.1.2.1). The fur looking excessively moist, even to drop when stretching out the tongue is named glossy fur (See color fig. 3.1.2.2). The fur looking dry and without fluid on it, even fissure is named dry fur (See color fig. 3.1.2.3). The dry coating without fluid on it, even rough like sands on it, is called rough coating (See color fig. 3.1.2.4).

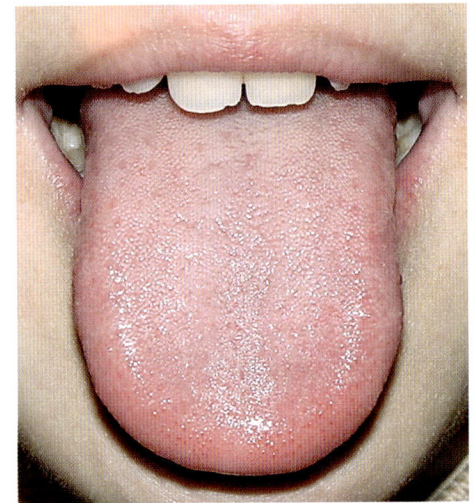

图(See color fig)3.1.2.1

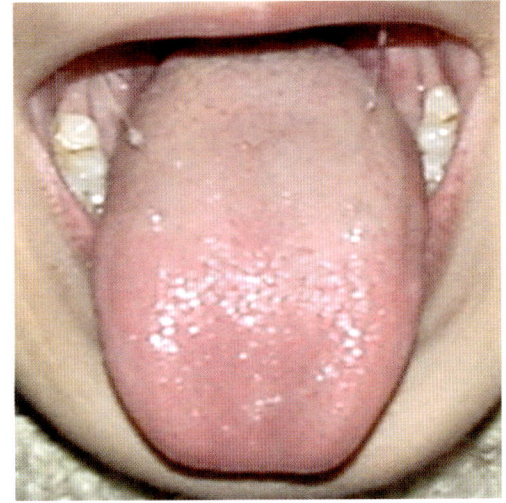

图(See color fig)3.1.2.2

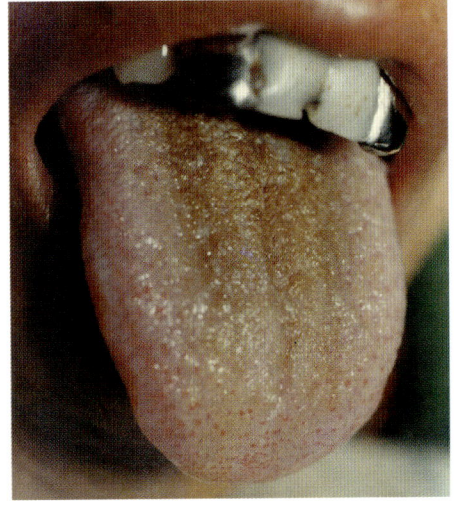

图(See color fig)3.1.2.3

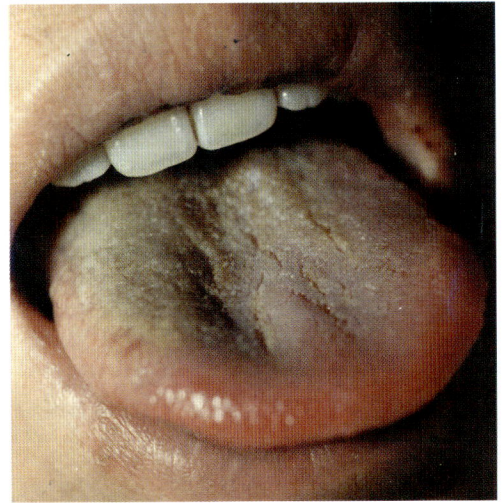

图(See color fig)3.1.2.4

润苔是正常舌苔的表现之一,是胃津、肾液上承,布露舌面所致。疾病过程中见润苔,提示体内津液未伤,如风寒表证、湿证初起、食滞、瘀血等均可见润苔(图 3.1.2.5)。

The well moisterized coating is taken as the normal condition. It results from plentiful fluid or stomach and kidney upward distribution on the surface of the tongue. The moist coating suggests that body fluid has not been impaired in the diseases such as the exterior syndromes of wind-cold, the early dampness syndromes, the retention of food and the blood stasis (See color fig. 3.1.2.5).

滑苔为水湿之邪内聚的表现,主痰饮、主湿。如寒湿内侵,或阳虚不能运化水液,寒湿、痰饮内生,都可出现滑苔(图 3.1.2.6)。

The glossy fur shows the existeance of *body-fluid* water-dampness retention. It often can be seen in phlegm or damp syndrome. It mostly results from invasion of cold-dampness into the interior or the retention of cold-dampness and phlegm which is due to deficient *yang* failing to promote water metabolism (See color fig. 3.1.2.6).

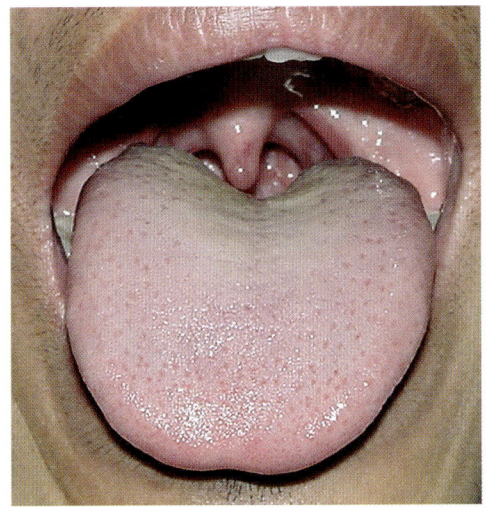

图(See color fig)3.1.2.5

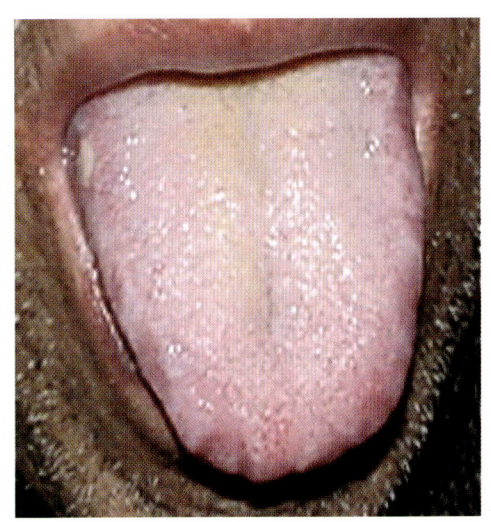

图(See color fig)3.1.2.6

燥苔提示体内津液已伤,如高热、大汗、吐泻后,或过服温燥药物等,导致津液不足,舌苔失于滋润而干燥(图 3.1.2.7)。亦有因痰饮、瘀血内阻,阳气被遏,不能上蒸津液濡润舌苔而见燥苔者,属津液输布障碍(图 3.1.2.8)、(图 3.1.2.9)。

The dry fur is due to injured body-dampness that results from high fever, excessive perspiration, and excessive vomiting and diarrhea or depletion of *yin* because of warm and dry drugs being used too much, which fail to moisturize the coating (See color fig. 3.1.2.7). It is also due to abnormal distribu-

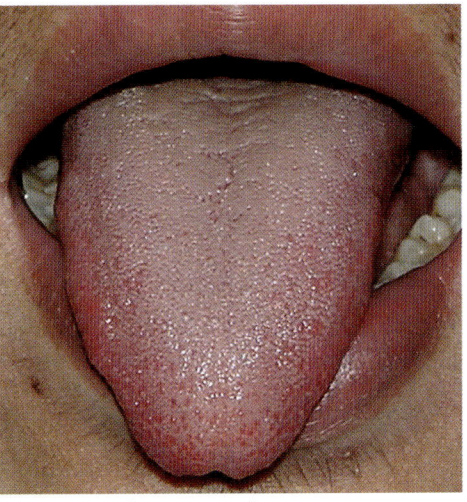

图(See color fig)3.1.2.7

tion of the body fluid resulting from the retention of phlegm, blood stasis or the obstacle from the retention of phlegm, blood stasis or the obstacle from *yang* failing to transform water into body fluid to moisturize the upper (See color fig. 3.1.2.8) (See color fig. 3.1.2.9).

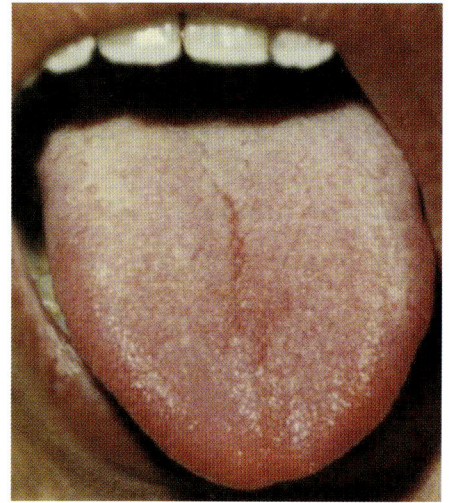
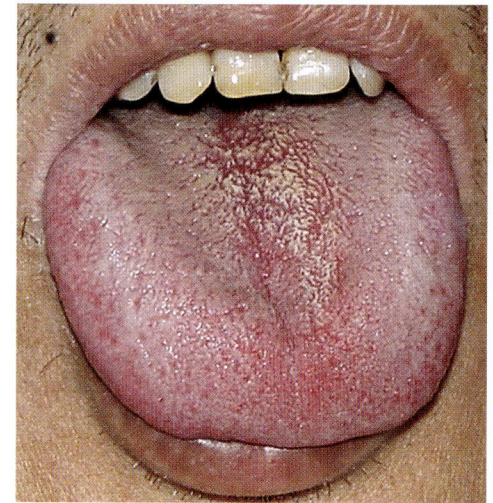

图(See color fig)3.1.2.8　　　　　　　　　图(See color fig)3.1.2.9

糙苔可由燥苔进一步发展而成。舌苔干结粗糙，津液全无，多见于热盛伤津之重证（图3.1.2.10）；苔质粗糙而不干者，多为秽浊之邪盘踞中焦（图3.1.2.11）。

The rough coating usually develops from the dry fur. The fur is rough and dry, without fluid on it, mostly can by seen in the serious symptoms of excessive heat impairing the body fluid (See color fig. 3.1.2.10). The fur is rough but not dry mostly results from retention of fetid evils in the *Middle-Jiao* (See color fig. 3.1.2.11).

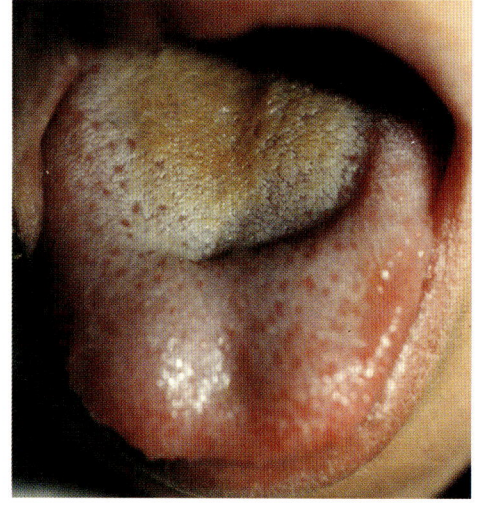
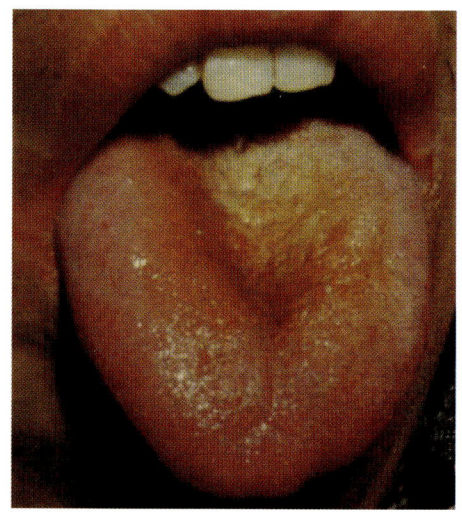

图(See color fig)3.1.2.10　　　　　　　　图(See color fig)3.1.2.11

舌苔由润变燥，表示热重津伤，或津失输布；舌苔由燥转润，主热退津复，或饮邪始化。故《辨舌指南》说:"滋润者其常,燥涩者其变;滋润者为津液未伤,燥涩者为津液已耗。"

The transformation of moist fur into dry fur suggest consumption of body fluid due to excessive heat or the body-fluid failing to distribute on the fur. The transformation of dry fur into moist fur indicates the setback of heat and the recovery of body fluid, or the transformation of the phlegm evils. *The guides for the tongue diagnosis* had said, "The moist coating is under the normal condition and the dry coating is under the abnormal condition. Moistness means the enough *body-fluid* and dryness shows exhaustion of the body-fluid."

此外,《察舌辨证新法》指出:"湿症舌润,热症舌燥,此理之常也。然亦有湿邪传入气分,气不化津而反燥者,热症传入血分,舌反润者……"说明舌苔的润、燥形成的机制不是单一的。

Besides, *New Methods of Differentiation of Deserving the Tongue* had said, "generally speaking, moistness suggests syndromes of dampness and dryness suggests syndromes of heat. However, some of the dry coating is not due to heat. When dampness enters into the *qi-phase* and makes failure of the *qi* in producing *body fluid*, dry coating may be seen. Some of the moist coating are also not due to cold, when warm-warm evils enter blood, it is a condition of the *yang* evils entering *yin* and making the *yin* streaming up, the coating becomes moist contrarily." All of the above shows that the theory of forming the moist fur or dry fur is not single.

3. 腻苔、腐苔
3. Putrid and Greasiness

苔质颗粒细腻致密,融合成片,中间厚边周薄,紧贴舌面,如油腻覆盖之状,揩之不去,刮之不脱,称为腻苔(图 3.1.3.1);苔质颗粒粗大疏松,形如豆腐渣堆积舌面,边中皆厚,揩之易去,称为腐苔(图 3.1.3.2)。若舌上黏厚一层,有如疮脓,则称脓腐苔(图 3.1.3.3)。

The compact and little grain-like fur, merging into pieces, thinner on the margin and thicker in the middle of the tongue surface, sticking on the surface tightly, and difficult to be scraped off, is named the greasy fur (See color fig. 3.1.3.1). It looks like being covered by greasy mucus. The loose and bigger grain-like fur, like the bean curd dregs

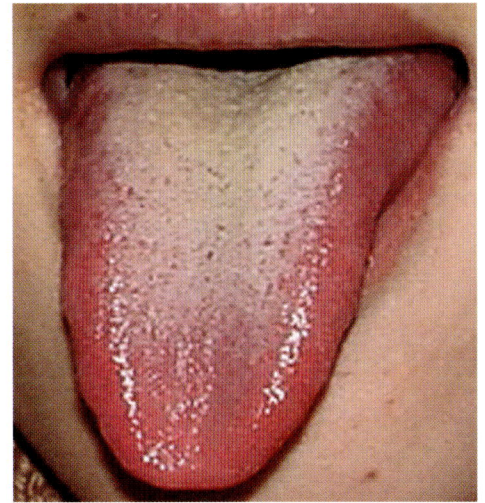

图(See color fig)3.1.3.1

heaped on the tongue surface, thicker in the margin and middle of the tongue surface, and easy to be scraped off, is named the putrid fur (See color fig. 3.1.3.2). The coating that looks like pus, thick and stick is named the pus-putrid coating (See color fig. 3.1.3.3).

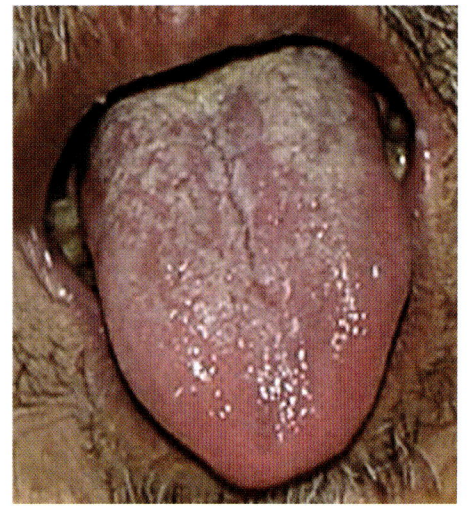

图(See color fig)3.1.3.2　　　　　　　图(See color fig)3.1.3.3

腻苔多由湿浊内蕴,阳气被遏,湿浊痰饮停聚舌面所致;腐苔多因阳热有余,蒸腾胃中秽浊之邪上泛,聚积舌面所致;脓腐苔,多见于内痈或邪毒内结,是邪盛病重的表现。

The greasy coating is a result of retention of pathogenic dampness and phlegm in the interior and on the tongue due to depression of *yang-qi*, on the other hand, the putrid coating usually results from the ascent of stale and turbid substances and pathogens in the stomach steamed by excessive yang-heat. The pus-putrid coating usually can be seen in the interior carbuncle and the combination of toxin and evils. It is a sign of excess evils and serious diseases.

舌苔薄腻,或腻而不板滞者,多为食积,或脾虚湿困,阻滞气机(图3.1.3.4);舌苔白腻而滑者,为痰浊、寒湿内阻,阳气被遏,气机阻滞(图3.1.3.5);舌苔粘腻而厚,口中发甜,是脾胃湿热,邪聚上泛(图3.1.3.6);舌苔黄腻而厚,为痰热、湿热、暑湿等邪内蕴,腑气不畅(图3.1.3.7)、(图3.1.3.8)。腐苔多为食积胃肠,或痰浊内蕴(图3.1.3.9)、(图3.1.3.10)。

The thin and greasy, or greasy but not sticky fur mostly suggests the retention of food, or the *yang* being encumbered by accu-

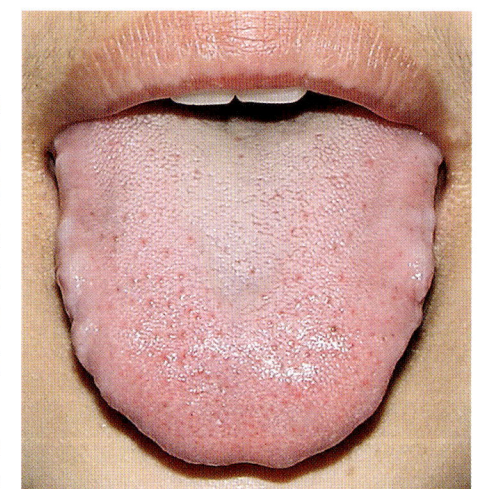

图(See color fig)3.1.3.4

mulated dampness inside, and the blocking of function of *qi* (See color fig. 3.1.3.4). If it is white, it is due to the retention of turbid-phlegm and cold-dampness, which encumbers the *yang-qi* and blocks the function of *qi* (See color fig. 3.1.3.5). If the coating is thick sticky and greasy, being accompanied by sweet taste in mouth, it is due to the raising upper by accumulated evils and damp-heat in the spleen and stomach (See color fig. 3.1.3.6). If the coating is yellow greasy and thick, it is due to the accumulation of evils of phlegm-heat, damp-heat or heat-dampness inside and unobstructed *bowel-qi* (See color fig. 3.1.3.7) (See color fig. 3.1.3.8). The putrid coating results from food-retention in the stomach and intestines or the stagnation of turbid-phlegm (See color fig. 3.1.3.9) (See color fig. 3.1.3.10).

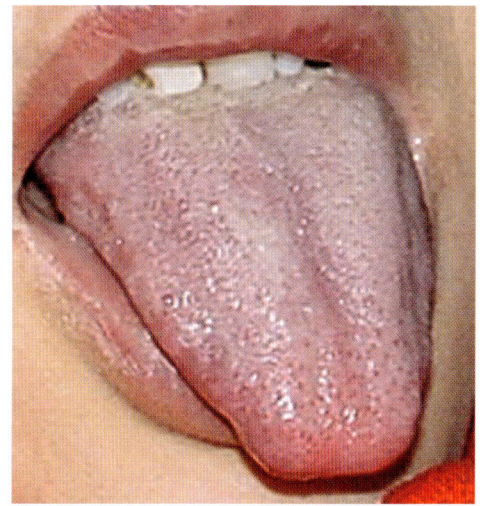

图(See color fig)3.1.3.5

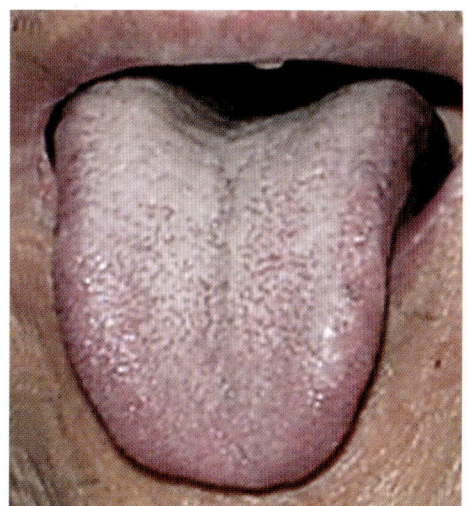

图(See color fig)3.1.3.6

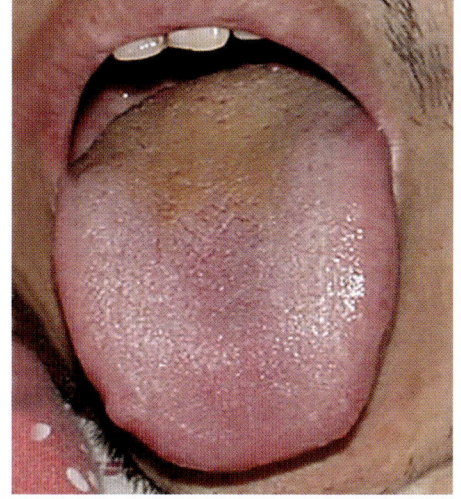

图(See color fig)3.1.3.7

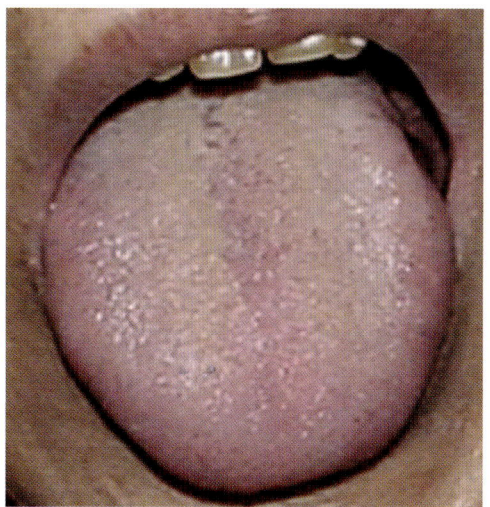

图(See color fig)3.1.3.8

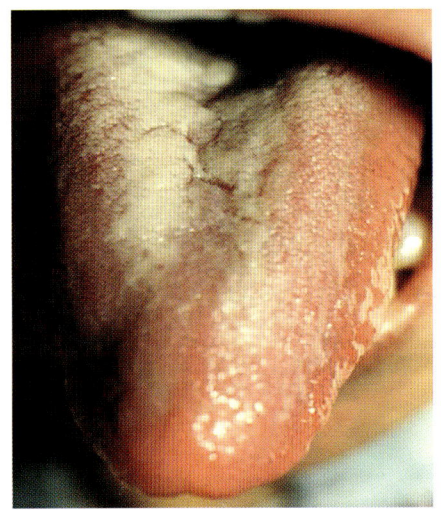 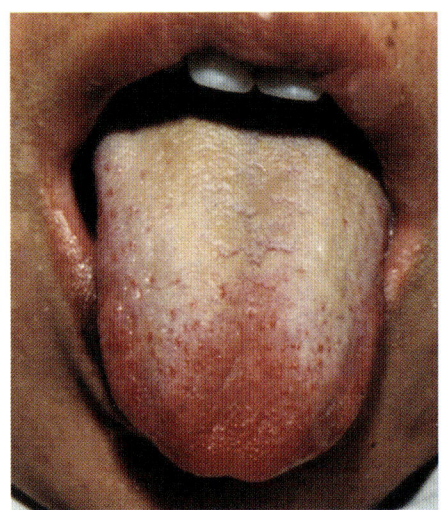

图(See color fig)3.1.3.9　　　　　　　图(See color fig)3.1.3.10

病中腐苔渐退,续生薄白新苔,为病邪消散,正气胜邪之象;若腐苔脱落,不能续生新苔者,为病久胃气衰败,正不胜邪之征。

If the putrid coating disappears slowly and the new thin white coating comes into being again, during the course of the disease, it is a sign of the vanish of evils and the evils being defeated by *geniune-qi*. If the putrid coating drops but the new coating can't form again, it is the sign of decline of *stomach-qi* or weakened *vital-qi* failing to defeat the evils.

4. 剥苔
4. Exfoliation

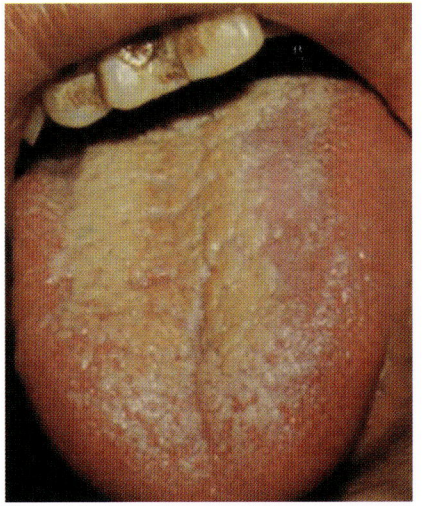

疾病过程中,舌苔全部或部分脱落,脱落处光滑无苔而可见舌质,称为剥苔(图 3.1.4.1)。多因胃气匮乏,不得上熏于舌,或胃阴枯涸,不能上潮于舌所致,亦是全身虚弱的一种征象。由于导致胃气、胃阴亏损的原因不同,损伤的程度亦有轻重,因而形成各种类型的剥脱苔。

If there is coating on tongue but no coating of some part or all coating disappears, where the texture of tongue can be seen, it is called exfoliation of coating (See color fig. 3.1.4.1). It mostly results from deficient *stomach-qi* failing to steam the tongue, or the exhaustion of stomach-yin failing to moisterize the tongue. It is also a sign of deficiency

图(See color fig)3.1.4.1

of the whole body. In general, exfoliate coating is formed as a result of impairment of both the *stomach-qi* and the *stomach-yin*, which therefore, exfoliate the fur.

根据舌苔剥脱的部位和范围大小不同,可分为以下几种:①舌前半部苔剥脱者,称前剥苔(图3.1.4.2),多为肺阴亏损;②舌中部苔剥脱者,称中剥苔(图3.1.4.3),多为脾胃亏虚;③舌根部苔剥脱者,称根剥苔(图3.1.4.4),多为肾阴枯竭;④舌苔多处剥脱,舌面仅斑驳残存少量舌苔者,称花剥苔(图3.1.4.5),多为邪实阴虚;⑤若剥脱处残存有腻苔者,多为正气亏虚,痰浊未化,病情较为复杂(图3.1.4.6);⑥舌苔周围剥脱,仅留中心一小块者,称为鸡心苔(图3.1.4.7),多为气血不足,阴血尤虚;⑦舌苔全部剥脱,舌面光洁如镜者,称为光剥苔或镜面舌(图3.1.4.8),多为胃乏生气之兆,属阴虚重证,为胃肾阴液枯竭;⑧舌苔不规则地剥脱,边缘凸起,界限清楚,形似地图,部位时有转移者,称为地图舌(图3.1.4.9),多见于儿童,与阴虚禀赋体质有关;⑨舌苔剥脱处,舌面不光滑,仍有新生苔质颗粒,或舌乳头可见者,称为类剥苔(图3.1.4.10),多为血虚或气血两虚,久病气血不续。

It can be divided into several kinds as follow. The coating exfoliates in the front half part of the tongue, which is named front exfoliate coating (See color fig. 3.1.4.2), suggests insufficient lung-*yin*. If the coating exfoliates in the middle of the tongue, it is named middle exfoliate coating and mostly indicates deficiency of spleen and stomach (See color fig. 3.1.4.3). If the coating exfoliates in the root of the tongue, it is name root exfoliate coating and usually means exhaustion of kidney-*yin* (See color fig. 3.1.4.4). If there is partial exfoliation of coating, and there is no coating at the exfoliated part, this is called versicolor exfoliate coating (tongue) (See color fig. 3.1.4.5). It mostly results from deficient *vital-qi* failing to prompt the turbid-phlegm, and the symptoms are more complicated (See color fig. 3.1.4.6). If there is partly exfoliating coating and only the center of the tongue surface coated is called chicken heart-like coating (See color fig. 3.1.4.7), which suggest deficient *qi* and blood, and deficient *yin-blood* especially. A furless tongue as smooth as a mirror is named mirror-like tongue or bare tongue (See color fig. 3.1.4.8), which suggest the exhaustion of *yin-fluid* in kidney and stomach. It is a sign of deficient active *qi* in stomach and belongs to serious syndromes in result of the deficiency of *yin*. The coating exfoliating irregularly, protruding on the margin, having clear boundary, looking like map and the location transferring here and there sometimes is name geographic tongue (See color fig. 3.1.4.9). It usually can be seen in children and is connected with the natural endowment of deficient *yin*. If the exfoliate part is somewhat rough and covered with new produced particle, on which the tongue mammilla can be seen, it is called "exfoliation-like tongue" (See color fig. 3.1.4.10). It mostly shows deficient blood of insufficient *qi* and blood, or discontinuation of the *qi* and blood because of long diseases.

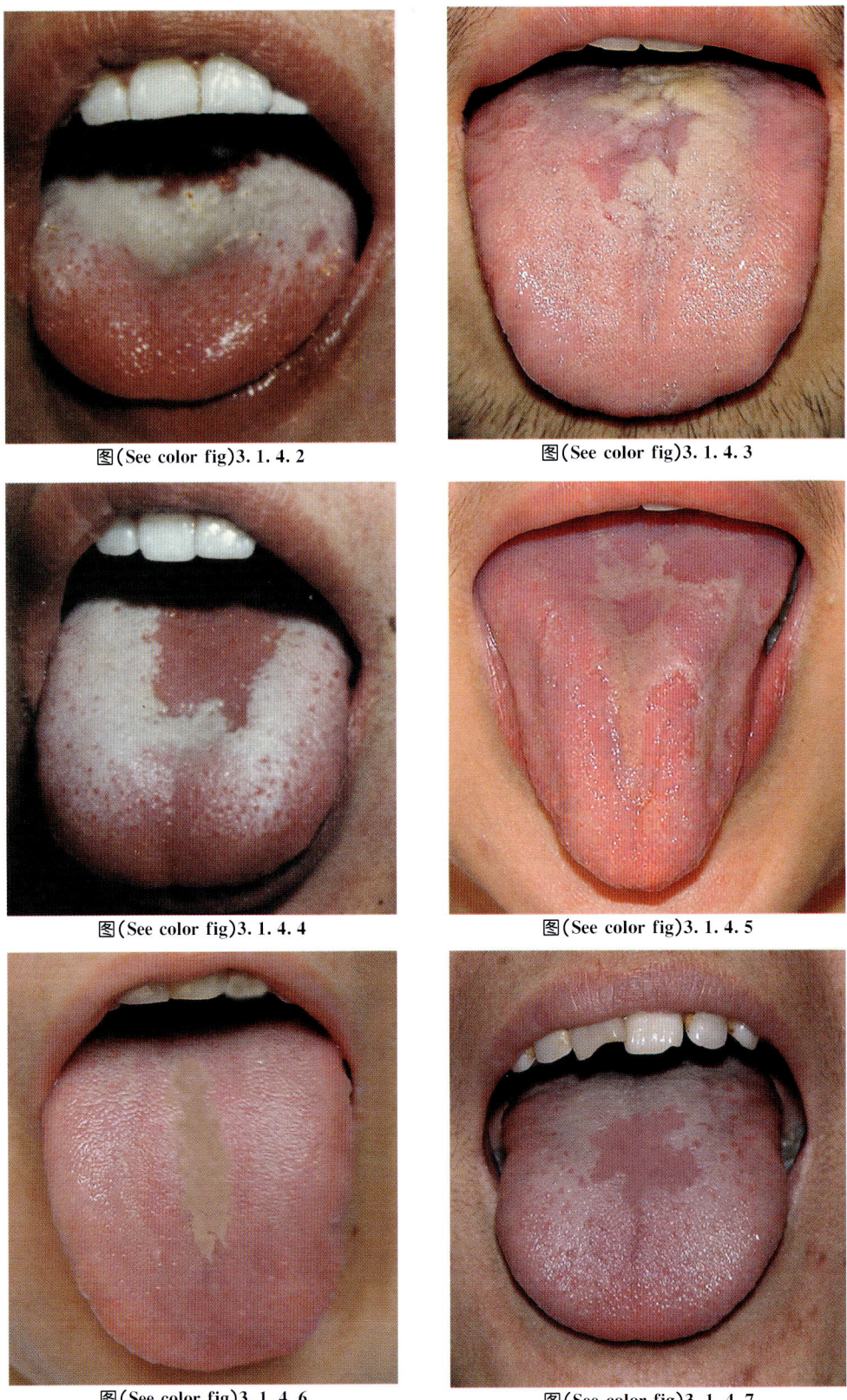

图(See color fig)3.1.4.2

图(See color fig)3.1.4.3

图(See color fig)3.1.4.4

图(See color fig)3.1.4.5

图(See color fig)3.1.4.6

图(See color fig)3.1.4.7

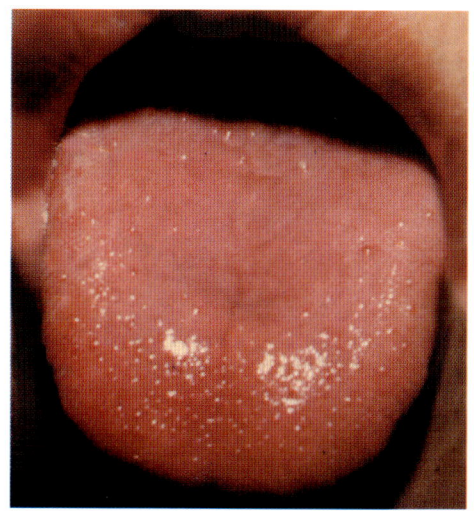
图(See color fig)3.1.4.8

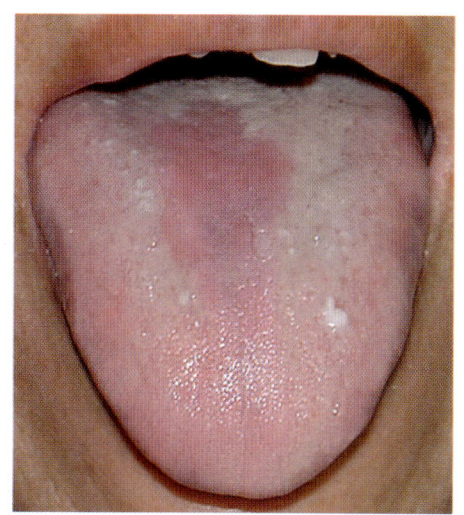
图(See color fig)3.1.4.9

总之,观察舌苔的有无、消长及剥脱变化,不仅能测知胃气、胃阴的存亡,亦可反映邪正盛衰,判断疾病的预后。如舌苔从全到剥,是胃的气阴不足,正气渐衰的表现;舌苔剥脱后,复生薄白之苔,为邪去正胜,胃气渐复之佳兆。

In general, observation of the exfoliate, wax and wane is helpful to distinguish the existence or the flee of the *stomach-qi* and stomach-yin, to reflect the exuberance or decline of the *genuine-qi*, and to judge the prognosis of the diseases. The change from the presence of fur to its absence is a manifestation of deficiency of *qi* and *yin* in stomach and gradual weakness of *vital qi*. On the contrary, the regeneration of a thin

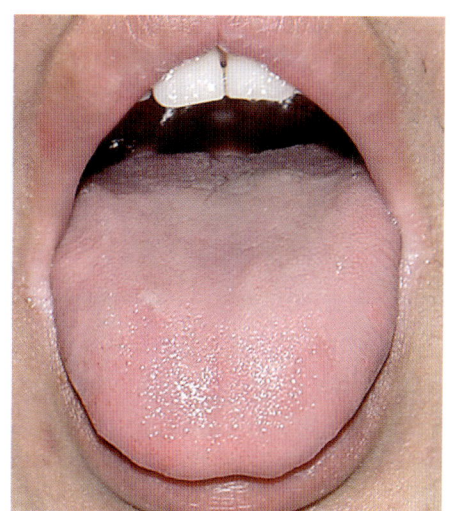
图(See color fig)3.1.4.10

and white coating after being stripped off is regarded as favorable sign of conquest of pathogens by *vital qi* and gradual recovery of the *stomach-qi*.

5. 偏苔、全苔
5. Evenness and Unevenness

舌苔遍布舌面,称为全苔(图3.1.5.1);舌苔仅布于前、后、左、右之某一局部,称为偏苔(图3.1.5.2)。病中见全苔,常主邪气散漫,多为湿痰阻滞之征。舌苔偏于某处,常示舌所分候的脏腑有邪气停聚。

The coating evenly spreading all over tongue surface is even coating (See color fig. 3.1.5.1). It is due to the over spreading evil, or the retention of damp-phlegm in diseases. If the coating is only on some parts of tongue surface, it is called uneven coating (See color fig. 3.1.5.2). The uneven coating may be on the front, rear, left, right part. The even coating on part that reflects the Zang-Fu suggests accumulation and retention of evils.

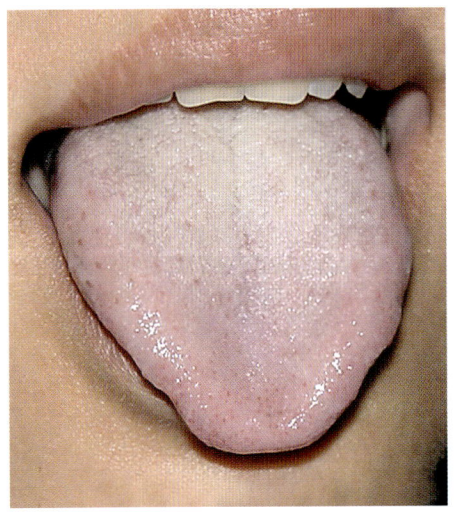

图(See color fig)3.1.5.1

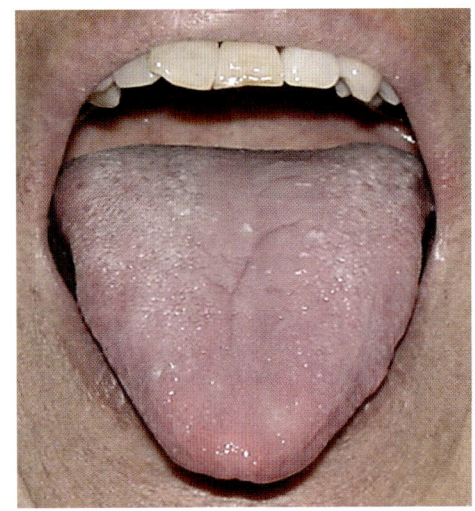

图(See color fig)3.1.5.2

舌苔偏于舌尖部,是邪气入里未深,而胃气却已先伤(图3.1.5.3);舌苔偏于舌根部,是外邪虽退,但胃滞依然(图3.1.5.4);舌苔仅见于舌中,常是痰饮、食浊停滞中焦(图3.1.5.5);舌苔偏于左或右,常提示肝胆湿热之类疾患(图3.1.5.6)。

The uneven coating on outer part (near the tip) is due to evil in the interior but not deep and the *stomach-qi* deficiency (See color fig. 3.1.5.3), that on inner part (near the root part) is due to the vanishing of exterior evil but heavy food retention in stomach (See color fig. 3.1.5.4). The uneven coating only on middle part is due to the retention of phlegm and food in *Middle-Jiao* (See color fig. 3.1.5.5). The even coating on one side, left or right, usually suggest evils of damp-heat in liver and gallbladder (See color fig. 3.1.5.6).

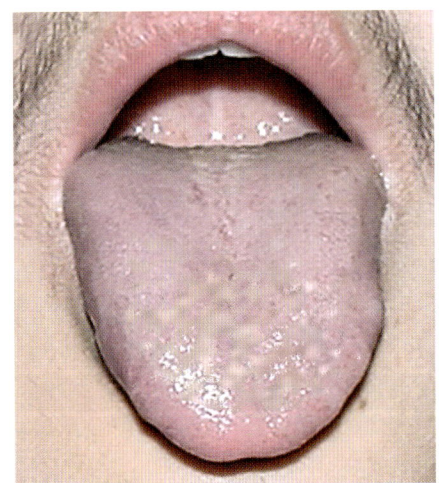

图(See color fig)3.1.5.3

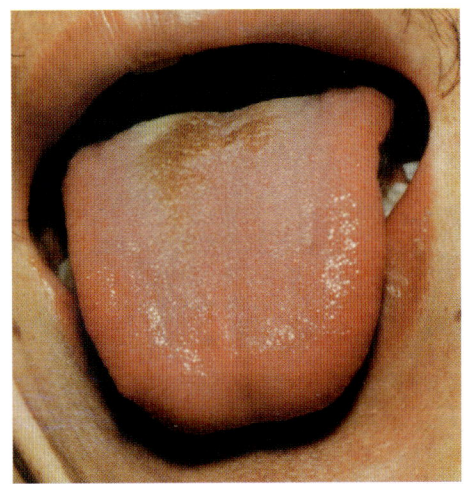

图(See color fig)3.1.5.4

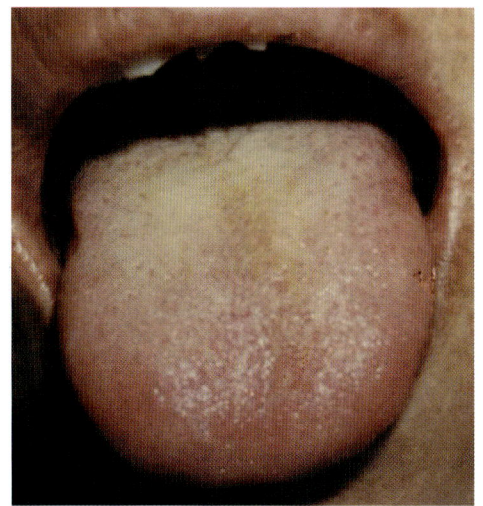
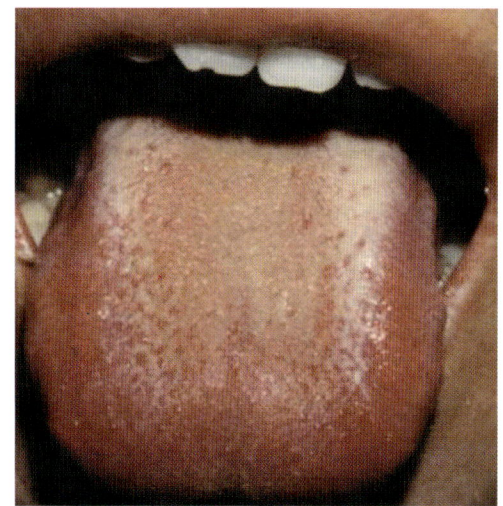

图(See color fig)3.1.5.5　　　　　　　　图(See color fig)3.1.5.6

偏苔应与剥苔相鉴别,偏苔为舌苔分布上的病理现象,并非剥苔之本来有苔而剥落,以致舌苔显示偏于某处。若因一侧牙齿脱落,摩擦减少而使该侧舌苔较厚者,与病理性偏苔有别。

The uneven coating should be distinguished from the exfoliate coating. The first is the pathological phenomena of coating distribution; the latter is original but exfoliated and results in uneven coating on somewhere. The coating being thicker on one side usually results from teeth lose and reduced friction , which should be differentiated from the pathological uneven coating.

6. 真苔、假苔
6. The True and False Coating

舌苔坚敛着实,紧贴于舌面,刮之难去,刮后仍留有苔迹,不露舌质,似从舌里长出者,称为真苔,即有根苔(图3.1.6.1);舌苔不紧贴舌面,似涂于舌面,苔易刮脱,刮后无垢而舌质光洁者,称为假苔,即无根苔(图3.1.6.2)。真苔是脾胃生气熏蒸食浊等邪气上聚于舌面而成,苔有根蒂,故舌苔与舌体不可分离。假苔是因胃气匮乏,不能续生新苔,而已生之旧苔逐渐脱离舌体,浮于舌面,故苔无根蒂,刮后无垢。

The true coating refers to the sturdy coating that is closely adhered to the tongue body and is difficult to be scraped off. The mark of the coating still remains after being scraped off, and the texture of the tongue is not exposed. It looks like growing out from the tongue body. It is also named rooted coating (See color fig. 3.1.6.1). The false coating is not closely adhered to the tongue body and is easy to be scraped off. It looks like being put on the tongue body. So the texture of the tongue is smooth and clear after the coating has been scraped off. It is also named non-rooted coating (See color fig. 3.1.6.2). The true coating is formed from the upper accumulation of evils such as turbid food steamed by the *spleen-qi* and *stomach-qi* on the surface of the tongue. The coating has root, so it can't be separated from the tongue body. The false coating is due to the deficient *stomach-qi* failing to produce new coating. But the old coating breaks away from the tongue body slowly and floats on the surface of the tongue. So the coating has no root and filth after being scraped off.

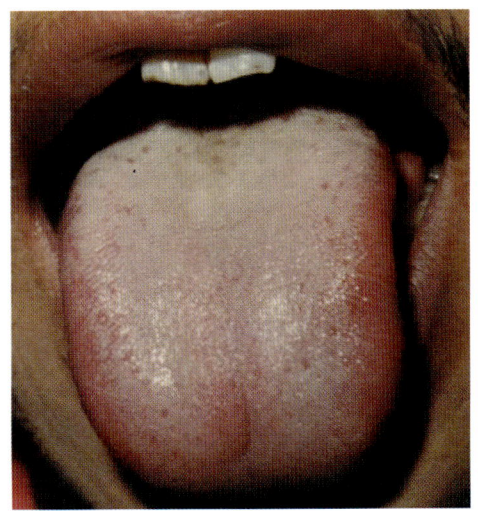
图(See color fig)3.1.6.1

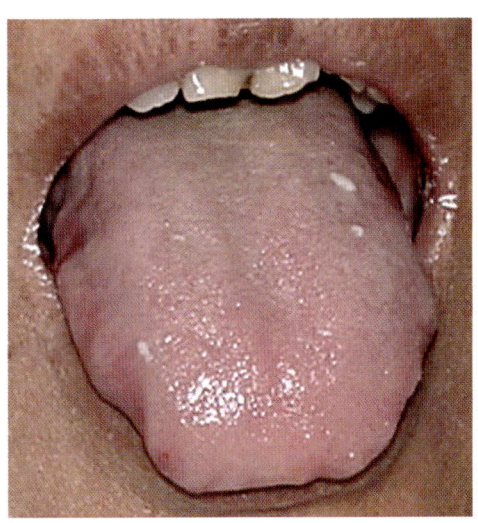
图(See color fig)3.1.6.2

辨苔之真假，对辨别疾病的轻重、预后有重要意义。病之初期、中期，舌见真苔且厚，为胃气壅实，病较深重；久病见真苔，说明胃气尚存。病出现假苔，是胃气匮乏，不能上潮，病情危重。舌面上浮一层厚苔，望似无根，刮后却见已有薄薄新苔者，是疾病向愈的善候。

To inspect whether the coating is true or false is important for judging the gravity of diseases and the goodness of the prognosis. The true and thick coating in the early and middle period of the disease, suggest jammed and excessive *stomach-qi* and more severe disease. The true coating can be seen also in the long period disease indicates the remains of *stomach-qi*. The false coating comes into being during the course of the disease that suggest deficient *stomach-qi* failing to tide up and the sign of dangerous diseases. Another condition of a layer of thick coating floating on the surface of the tongue and looked like non-rooted, and thin new-produced coating below it after being scraped off is a good omen of recovery.

第二节 诊 苔 色
Section 2 Color of Tongue Coating

根据舌苔的颜色，舌苔分白、黄、灰黑苔几类，临床可单独出现，亦可相兼出现。

There are whit, yellow, gray and black colors of coating. They may come into being in single or in combination.

1. 白苔
1. White Coating

舌面上所附着的苔垢呈现白色,称为白苔(图 3.2.1.1),白苔有厚薄之分,苔白而薄,透过舌苔可看到舌体者,是薄白苔(图 3.2.1.2);苔白而厚,不能透过舌苔见到舌体者,是厚白苔(图 3.2.1.3)。白舌苔为苔之本色,正常人多为薄白苔,在疾病中出现多见于表证、寒证、湿证,亦可见于热证,其他苔色均可由白苔转化而成。

The coating being adhered to the surface of the tongue in white color is named white coating (See color fig. 3.2.1.1). It can be divided into thick white and thin white coating, and through which the tongue body can be seen (See color fig. 3.2.1.2). The thick white coating refers to white and thick coating

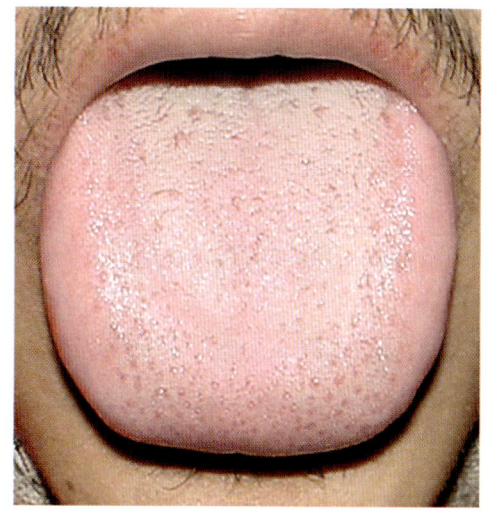

图(See color fig)3.2.1.1

(See color fig. 3.2.1.3), and through which the tongue body can't be seen white is the natural color of the coating. It is a sign of normal condition, and usually can be seen during the diseases of exterior syndromes, cold syndromes, damp syndromes and heat syndromes. The other color coating all may be transformed from the white coating.

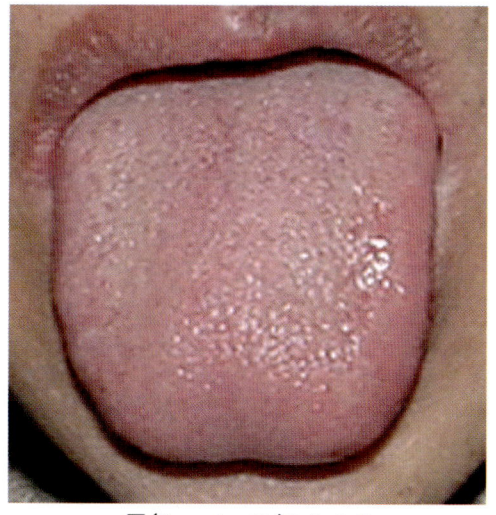

图(See color fig)3.2.1.2

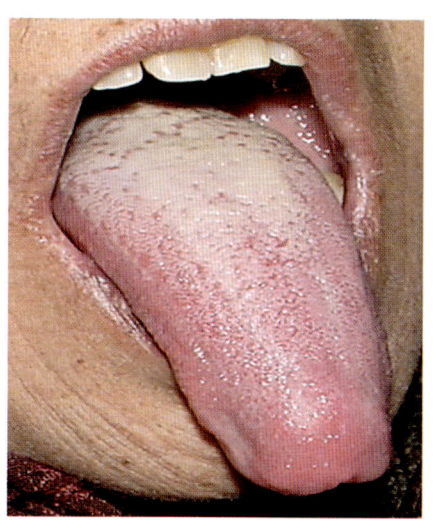

图(See color fig)3.2.1.3

苔薄白而润,可为正常舌象,或为表证初起,或是里证病轻,或是阳虚内寒(图 3.2.1.4);苔薄白而滑,多为外感寒湿,或脾肾阳虚,水湿内停(图 3.2.1.5);苔薄白而干,多由外感风热所致(图 3.2.1.6);苔白厚腻,多为中阳不振,湿浊痰饮内停,或肠胃食积停滞(图 3.2.1.7);苔白厚而干,主痰浊湿热内蕴(图 3.2.1.8);苔白如积粉,扪之不燥者,称为积粉苔,常见于瘟疫或内痈等病,系秽浊湿邪与热毒相结而成(图 3.2.1.9);苔白而燥裂,粗糙如砂石,提示燥热伤津,阴液亏损(图 3.2.1.10)。

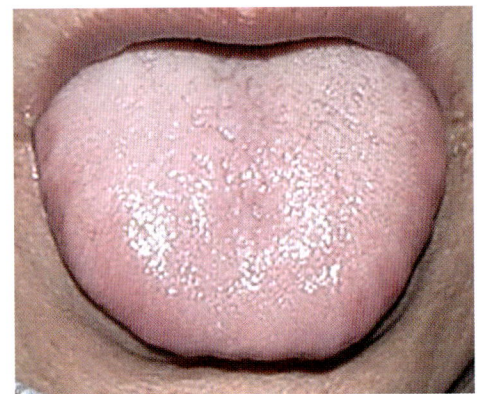

图(See color fig)3.2.1.4

The thin, white and moist coating may be under normal condition or suggests the beginning of the exterior syndromes, or the light or shallow interior syndromes, or the interior cold resulting from deficient *yang* (See color fig. 3.2.1.4). The thin, white and slippery coating is mostly due to the exterior cold-dampness, or internal retention of water-dampness caused by deficient *spleen-yang* and *kidney-yang* (See color fig. 3.2.1.5). The thin, white and dry coating is usually due to the exterior wind-heat (See color fig. 3.2.1.6). The white, thick and greasy coating often results from the internal retention of turbid dampness and phlegm caused by uninspired *Middle-Yang*, or the retention of food in the stomach and intestines (See color fig. 3.2.1.7). The thick, white and dry coating indicates the internal accumulation of phlegm and damp-heat (See color fig. 3.2.1.8). The white coating spreading over the tongue like the heaped powder, but not being dry while palpated is called the powder-like coating, as a result of the combination of the filthy and turbid dampness with the heat toxin (See color fig. 3.2.1.9). It is often seen in pestilence and abscess of internal organs. The white and dry fur like sand, being rough while palpated, suggests the damaged body fluid by dry-heat and the exhaustion of *yin-fluid* (See color fig. 3.2.1.10).

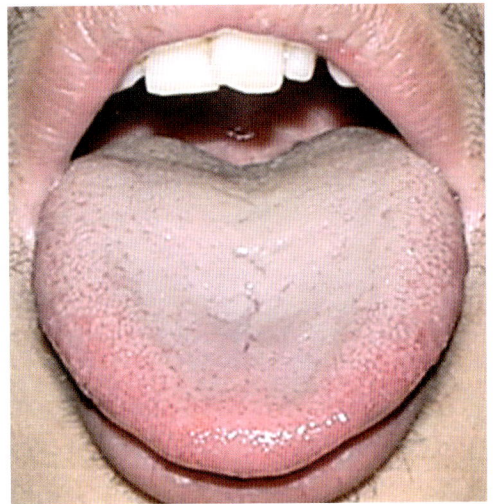

图(See color fig)3.2.1.5

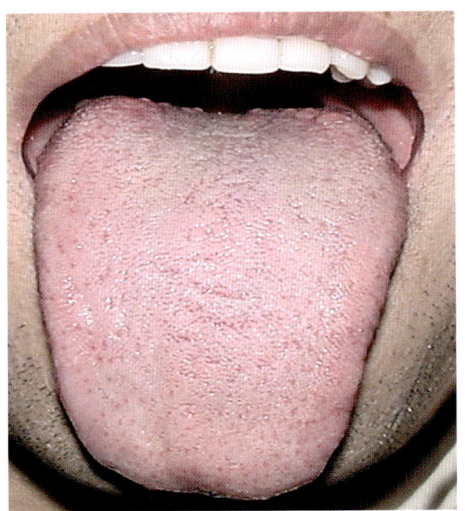

图(See color fig)3.2.1.6

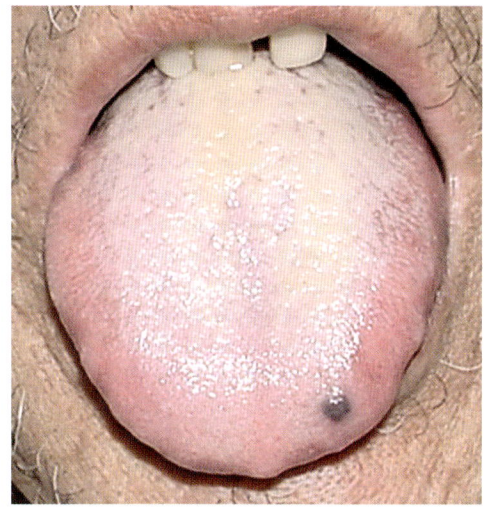

图(See color fig)3.2.1.7

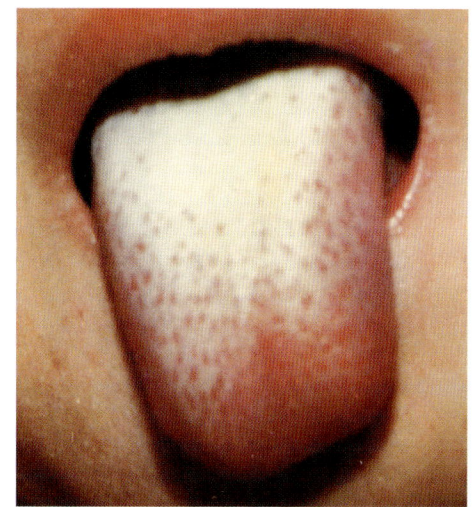

图(See color fig)3.2.1.8

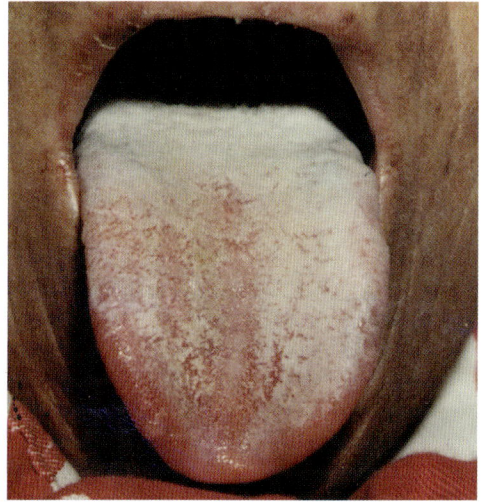

图(See color fig)3.2.1.9

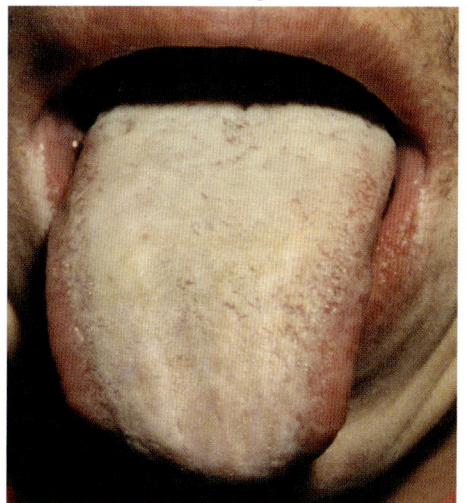

图(See color fig)3.2.1.10

2. 黄苔
2. The Yellow Coating

舌面上所附着的苔垢呈现黄色,称为黄苔(图3.2.2.1)。据苔黄的程度,有淡黄、深黄和焦黄之分。淡黄又称微黄苔,是指舌苔呈浅黄色(图3.2.2.2);深黄又称正黄苔,是指舌苔黄而深厚(图3.2.2.3);焦黄又称老黄,是指舌苔呈现黄黑色(图3.2.2.4)。黄苔多因感受热邪或病邪入里化热,邪热熏灼于舌所致。故一般而论,苔呈黄色,苔色愈黄,说明热邪愈甚;淡黄苔为热轻,深黄苔为热甚,焦黄苔为热极。黄苔多分布于舌中,亦可布满全舌,多与红、绛舌同时出现。黄苔还有厚薄、润燥、腻等苔质变化。

If the coating being adhered to the surface of the tongue is yellow in color, it called yellow coating (See color fig. 3.2.2.1). It can be divided into light yellow, heavy yellow and brown yellow coating. The light yellow coating, also being named minute yellow coating, is referred that the coating that is light yellow color (See color fig. 3.2.2.2). The heavy yellow coating, also called right yellow coating, is referred that the coating that is thick and yellow in color (See color fig. 3.2.2.3). The black yellow coating is called brown coating, which is called tough yellow coating (See color fig. 3.2.2.4). The yellow coating mostly results from the invasion of heat evils, or the evil from the exterior into the interior producing heat and the heat evils stifling on the tongue. In generally speaking, the degree of yellow of the coating is related to the degree of heat. The deeper the yellow of the tongue coating, the more intense the pathogenic heat. The light yellow coating suggests shallow heat, while heavy yellow coating deep heat and brown yellow coating extremely excessive heat. The yellow coating mostly distributes in the middle of the tongue, also spreads over the whole tongue. It usually comes into being with the red and crimson tongue. The yellow coating has changes of thick and thin, moist and dry, greasy tongue texture etc also.

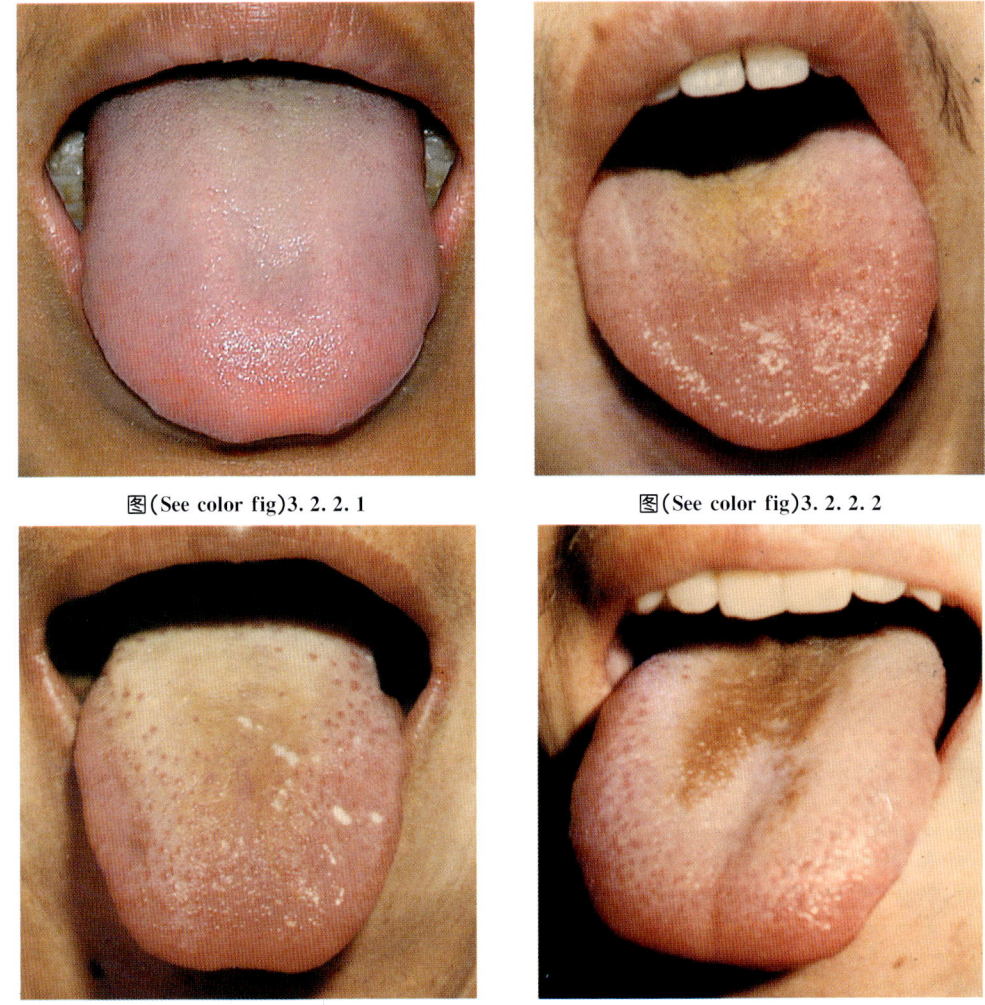

图(See color fig)3.2.2.1

图(See color fig)3.2.2.2

图(See color fig)3.2.2.3

图(See color fig)3.2.2.4

舌苔由白转黄,或呈黄白相兼,为外感表证处于化热入里,表里相兼阶段。故《伤寒指掌》说:"白苔主表,黄苔主里,太阳主表,阳明主里,故黄苔专主阳明里证。辨证之法,但看舌苔带一分白,病亦带一分表,必纯黄无白,邪方离表入里。"

The changing of coating colors from white to yellow or to combined white and yellow suggests the exterior evils into the interior and producing heat, or the stage of combination exterior and interior syndromes. So *Finger and Palm of Cold-Attack* said, "The white coating indicates exterior syndromes while yellow coating interior syndromes. *Tai-Yang* controls the exterior while *Yang-Ming* the interior. So, the yellow coating suggests the interior syndromes in *Yang-Ming*. In exogenous disease, the white coating means the disease is in the exterior. The yellowish white coating means the disease is partially in both interior and exterior. If the coating is purely yellow without any white, it is the emblem of all evils in the interior.

苔色淡黄,苔质较薄者,为风热之邪犯表或风寒郁遏化热火里(图3.2.2.5);苔色深黄,为里热夹湿,或痰饮化热,或食积热腐(图3.2.2.6);苔色焦黄,为里热伤津,燥结腑实(图3.2.2.7)。

The light yellow and thin coating indicates invasion by exogenous wind-heat or heat transformed from obstacle wind-cold entering the interior (See color fig. 3.2.2.5). The heavy yellow coating suggests the internal heat carrying dampness, or heat transformed from phlegm, or the retention of food rotted by the heat (See color fig. 3.2.2.6).

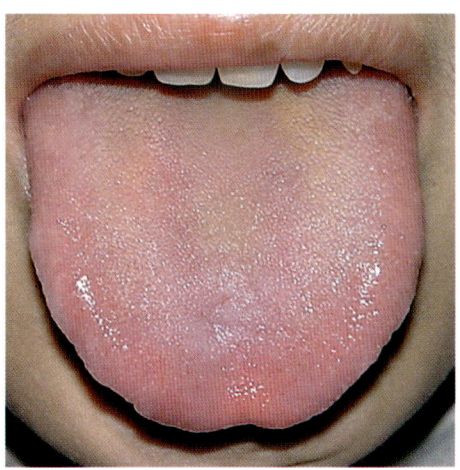

图(See color fig)3.2.2.5

The coating in brown yellow results from the impaired body fluid caused by internal heat or bound dryness and the excessive syndromes in bowels (See color fig. 3.2.2.7).

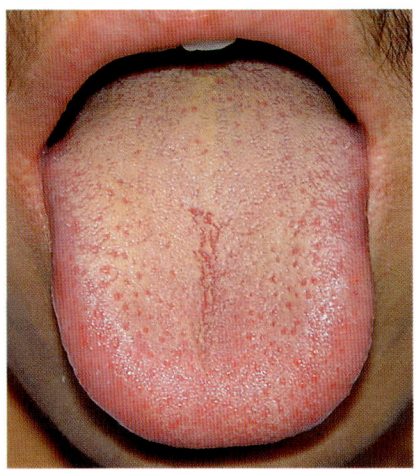

图(See color fig)3.2.2.6

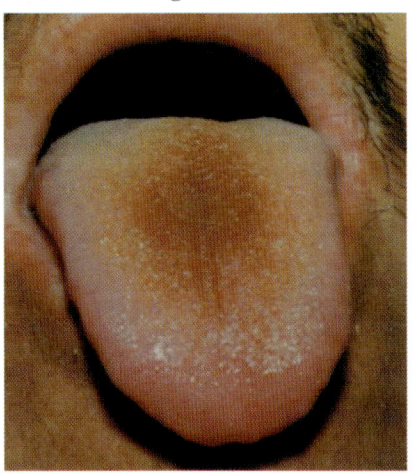

图(See color fig)3.2.2.7

苔淡黄而润滑多津者,称为黄滑苔(图3.2.2.8),多为阳虚寒湿之体,痰饮聚久化热;或为气血亏虚复感湿热之邪所致。黄苔而质腻者,称黄腻苔(图3.2.2.9),主湿热或痰热内蕴,或为食积化腐。苔黄黑质粘腻者,为霉酱苔(图3.2.2.10);多由胃肠素有湿浊宿食,积久化热,熏蒸秽浊上泛舌面所致,亦可见于湿热夹痰的病证。

The yellow slippery coating is so named because the coating is moist, slippery, light yellow in color and with much fluid on the tongue surface (See color fig. 3.2.2.8). It mostly results from deficient *yang* and cold-dampness in nature, or heat transformed from

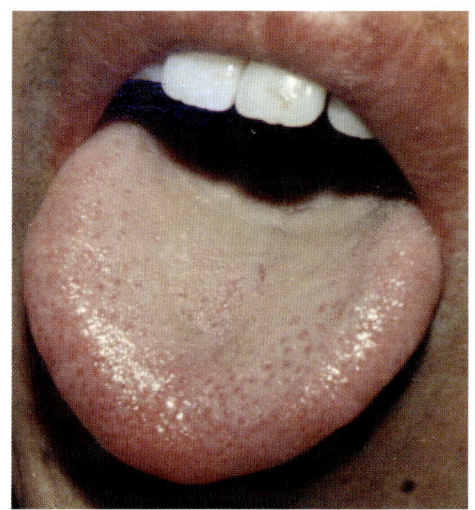

图(See color fig)3.2.2.8

the long accumulated phlegm, or the re-attack of damp-heat evils on the body with insufficient *qi* and blood. If the color of coating is yellow and the texture of the coating is grease. It is named the yellow greasy coating (See color fig. 3.2.2.9). It suggests the internal accumulation of damp-heat or phlegm-heat, or the retention of food rotten by heat. The coating texture is named mould sauce coating (See color fig. 3.2.2.10). It is usually due to the turbid dampness and old food, being accumulated too long and transformed into heat, which steams the filthy-turbid upward on the surface of the tongue. It also can be seen in the syndromes of damp-heat carrying phlegm.

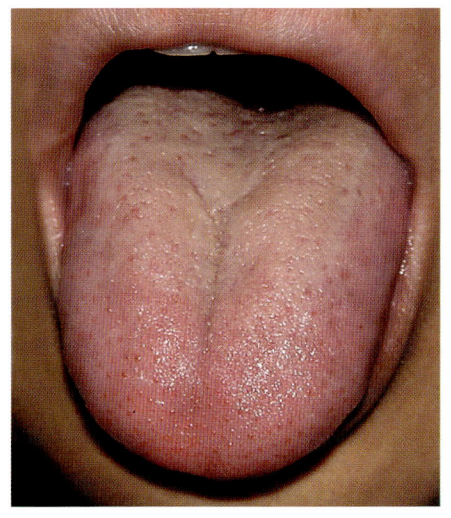

图(See color fig)3.2.2.9

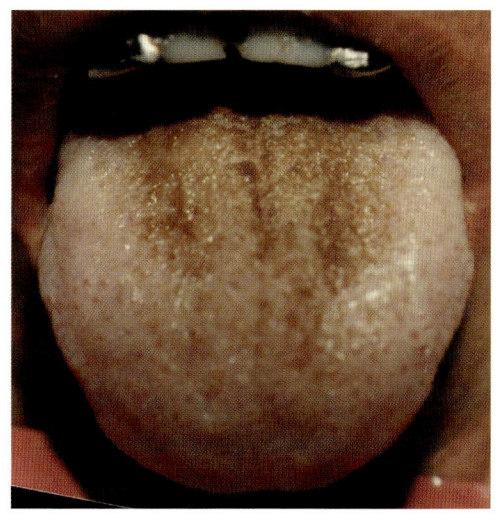

图(See color fig)3.2.2.10

苔黄而干燥,甚至苔干而硬,颗粒粗大,扪之糙手者,称黄糙苔(图3.2.2.11);苔黄而干涩,中有裂纹如花瓣状,称黄瓣苔(图3.2.2.12);黄黑相兼,如烧焦的锅巴,称焦黄苔

(图 3.2.2.13)。均主邪热伤津,燥结腑实之证。

The coating being dry and yellow in color, even dry and stiff with rough and big particles, and rough while palpated, is named yellow rough coating (See color fig. 3.2.2.11). The dry and yellow coating, with fissures like petals in the middle, is named yellow petal coating (See color fig. 3.2.2.12). Combined yellow and black coating, that looks like the rice crust burnt and charred, is called brown coating (See color fig. 3.2.2.13). Both suggest the impaired body fluid because of heat evils and syndromes of bund dryness and bowel-excess.

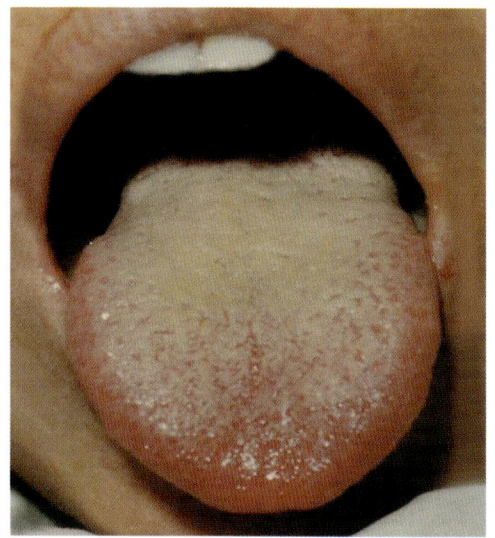

图(See color fig)3.2.2.11

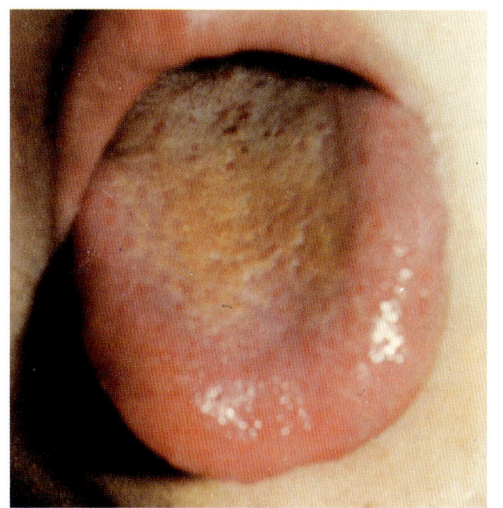

图(See color fig)3.2.2.12

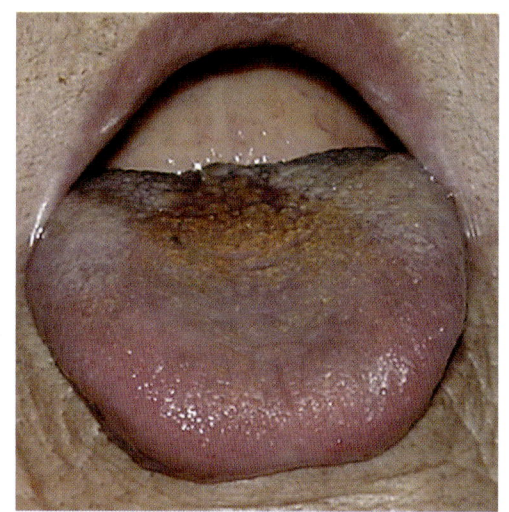

图(See color fig)3.2.2.13

3. 灰苔、黑苔
3. The Gray and Black Coating

苔色浅黑,称为灰苔(图 3.2.3.1);苔色深灰,称为黑苔(图 3.2.3.2)。灰苔与黑苔,只是颜色深浅之差别,故并称为灰黑苔。灰黑苔多由白苔或黄苔转化而成,多在疾病持续一定时日、发展到相当程度后才出现。灰黑苔可见于寒湿病中,亦可见于热性病中,多因阴寒内盛、或里热炽盛所致。

The gray coating means that the coating is light black in color (See color fig.

3.2.3.1). The black coating is named so because of the coating being in deep gray color (See color fig. 3.2.3.2). The gray coating and black coating only has difference in light or deep color and is always called as gray-black coating. It is mostly transformed from the white or yellow coating. It often comes into being while the disease have remained some days and developed to considerable extent. The gray-black coating may be seen in the disease of cold-dampness, and hot nature also. It mostly results from the excessive internal *yin*-cold and heat.

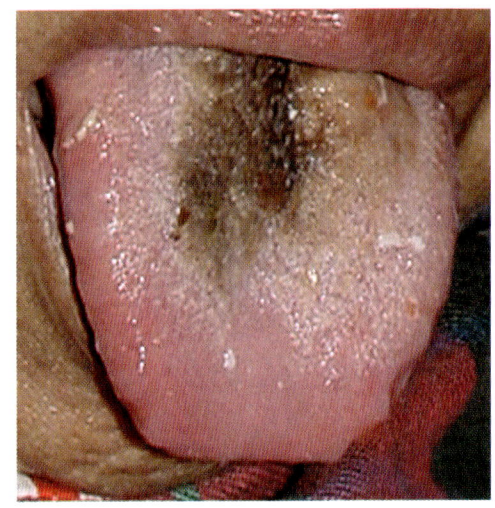
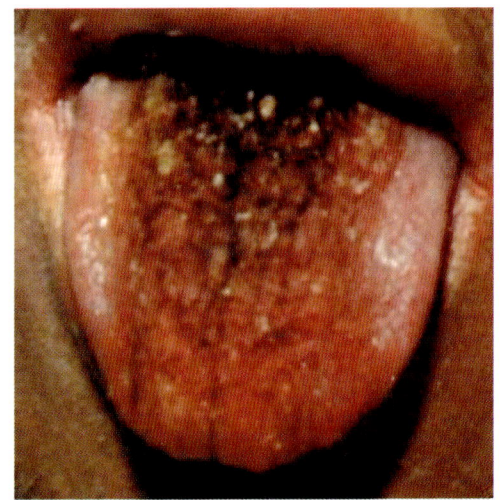

图(See color fig)3.2.3.1　　　　　　图(See color fig)3.2.3.2

　　无论寒热均属重证，黑色越深，病情越重。如《敖氏伤寒金镜录》说："舌见黑色，水克火明矣，患此者百无一治。"又说："若见舌胎如黑漆之光者，十无一生。"但亦有苔灰黑而病轻，甚至无明显症状者，如吸烟过多者，可见舌苔灰黑。

　　The black coating usually appears in the critical stage of disease, indicating either cold or heat in nature. The deeper the black of the coating, the more severe the disease is. Just as *Ao's Records of Golden Mirror on Cold Attack* had said that, "The black coating indicates that the fire light has been restricted by water. None of the patients with black coating could be cured." and had said again, "None of the patient with black coating likes black lacquer could be survived." The gray-black coating does not absolutely suggest the critical case. It also suggests shallow disease and even no symptoms. It can be cause by too much smoking.

　　苔质的润燥是辨别灰黑苔寒热属性的重要指征，在寒湿病中出现灰黑苔，多由白苔转变而成，其舌苔灰黑必湿润多津(图3.2.3.3)；在热性病中出现，多由黄苔转变而来，其舌苔灰黑必干燥无津液(图3.2.3.4)。

　　Moistness and dryness of coating texture is the important index for the clinical doctor to judge the gray-black coating resulting from wither cold or heat. The gray-black coating in disease of cold-dampness is mostly transformed from white coating. It should be moist and with much fluid on the surface (See color fig. 3.2.3.3). The gray-black coating in cases of hot nature is usually transformed from the yellow coating. It should be dry and with no fluid on the surface (See color fig. 3.2.3.4).

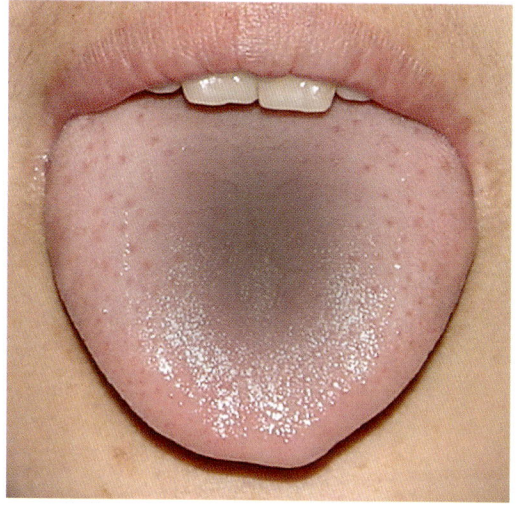
图(See color fig)3.2.3.3

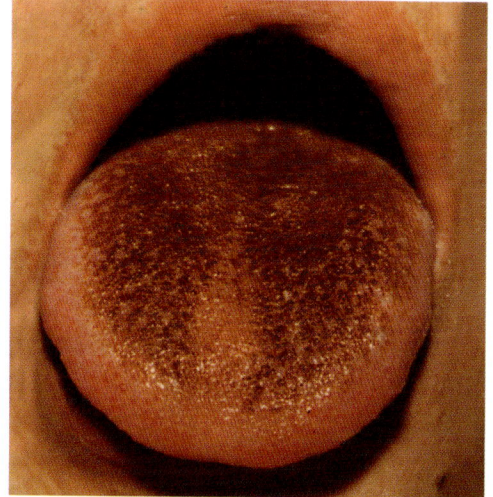
图(See color fig)3.2.3.4

舌边舌尖部呈白腻苔,而舌中和舌根部出现灰黑苔,舌面湿润,为阳虚寒湿内盛,或痰饮停聚;舌尖舌边黄腻苔,而舌中为灰黑苔,为湿热内阻,日久不化;苔焦黑干燥,舌质干裂起刺,不论是外感或是内伤病,均为热极津枯之征。

The white greasy coating being on the margin and tip, and gray-black being on the middle and root of the tongue with moisture suggests the deficient yang and internal excessive cold-dampness, or the retention and accumulation of phlegm. Yellow greasy coating on the tip and margin and gray-black coating on the middle of the tongue suggests the internal obstacle of damp-heat, which has not be resolved for a long time. The dry brown coating, whether in exogenous or endogenous disease, is a manifestation of extreme heat and exhaustion of body fluid.

第四章 舌诊的临床意义及应用

Chapter 4 The Usage and Significance of Tongue Inspection

《临症验舌法》指出:"凡内外杂证,无一不呈其形、著其气于舌,……据舌以分虚实,而虚实不爽焉;据舌以分阴阳,而阴阳不谬焉;据舌以分脏腑、配主方,而脏腑不差、主方不误焉。危急疑难之顷,往往无证可参、脉无可按,而惟以舌为凭;妇女幼稚之病,往往闻之无息,问之无声,而惟有舌可验。"可见,舌象诊断不仅意义普遍,而且客观准确、简便易行,故成为中医辨证的常规手段和重要依据。

Methods of Tongue Inspection in Clinic says, "Neither the exogenous nor the interior injured syndromes can not be reflected by the changes of shape, size, color, vitality and movement of the tongue. If we distinguish the deficiency from the excess in according to the tongue, the deficiency and excess would not be wrong. If we judge *yin* and *yang* in the light of the tongue, *yin* and *yang* wouldn't be mistaken. If we detect the location of disease in viscera and match the major prescription on the basis of the tongue, the location and the prescription would not be in error. Only the tongue can be depended on when the disease is severe and difficult to differentiate, or there are usually no symptoms to be consulted and no pulse to be palpated. The disease of female and children patients, often showing no information with auscultation and olfaction, or no answer with interrogation, only rely on the changes of the tongue". It is shown that, the significance of tongue inspection is not only universal, but also objective and accurate. The methods of tongue inspection are simple and convenient. So, it becomes the conventional means and important basis of differentiation in TCM.

第一节 舌诊的临床意义
Section 1 Significance of Tongue Inspection

舌象的变化能较客观准确的反映病情,可作为诊断疾病、了解病情的发展变化和辨证的重要依据。

The changes of tongue reflect the state of an illness objectively and exactly. They can be regarded as important basis for diagnosing diseases, understanding the development and changes of the state of an illness, and differentiation.

1. 判断邪正盛衰
1. To judge the exuberance or decline of the *vital-qi* and the *pathogenic-qi*

邪气与正气之盛衰,可在舌象方面反映出来。如舌有神者正气旺,舌少神者正气弱,舌无神者正气败;舌体淡红,柔软灵活,苔薄白而润,说明正气充足,气血运行正常,津液末未伤;舌色淡白,是气血两虚;舌干苔燥,是津液已伤;舌苔有根,是胃气充足;舌苔无根或光剥无苔,是胃气衰败;舌苔厚则为邪气盛,舌苔薄则为邪气不盛。

The exuberance or decline of the *vital-qi* and the *pathogenic-qi* can be shown in tongue. The tongue full of vitality suggests sufficient vital-qi, while lack of vitality insufficient vital-qi. The soft and flexible tongue in pink color with thin, white and moist coating indicates sufficient vital-qi, the normal moving of qi and blood, and the uninjured body fluid. The tongue white in color usually results from the deficiency of both qi and blood. The dry tongue and coating is due to the impairment of body fluid. The rooted coating means sufficient stomach-qi, while the non-rooted or whole exfoliated coating is usually caused by the declined *stomach-qi*. The thick coating suggests flourishing *pathogenic-qi*, while thin coating non-flourishing *pathogenic-qi*.

2. 区别病邪性质
2. To distinguish the nature or disease

不同性质的邪气致病,在舌象上会反映出不同的变化。一般而言,外感风寒,苔多薄白;外感风热,苔多薄黄;寒湿为病,多舌胖苔腻;燥邪为患,多舌红苔干;火热内盛,多舌红苔黄燥;痰浊内阻,苔多粘腻,水饮停聚,苔多水滑;食滞内停,苔多粗腐;另外,虫积者,舌可见凹陷圆红点;瘀血者,舌多见紫暗斑点;中毒者,舌可显蓝色。故风、寒、热、湿、燥、火、痰、饮、水、食、瘀、虫等诸种病因,大多可从舌象上加以鉴别。

Evils of different natures will make different changes of the tongue. In general speaking, the thin and white coating mostly results from exogenous wind-cold, while thin and yellow coating often results from exogenous wind-heat. The enlarged and fat tongue with greasy coating on the surface is usually due to the retention of cold-dampness. The tongue in red color with dry coating is always caused by the attack of dry evils. The interior flourishing fire-heat often results in red tongue and dries, yellow coating. The internal retention of phlegm-turbid usually leads to sticky and greasy coating. The slippery coating, with much fluid on the surface, is mostly caused by the retention of water-phlegm. The rough and putrid coating indicates the food-retention. Besides the above all, the sunken, round and red spots on the tongue body may be seen in patients with parasitic diseases. Dark purple spots on the tongue body mostly result from the blood stasis. The tongue may show bluish color among the persons with intoxication. So, all kinds of pathogenic wind, cold, heat, dampness, dryness, fire, phlegm, water, food, blood stasis and parasitic, mostly can be distinguished from the changes of the tongue.

3. 判别病位浅深
3. To detect the shallow or deep location of disease

病位的变化在舌象上也有相应的表现。舌苔与舌体候病有浅深侧重之分,舌体部位候病又有脏腑分属之别,故大体而言,病邪轻浅,多见舌苔变化,而病情深重可见舌质、舌苔同时变化。如外感病中,苔薄白是疾病初起,病情轻浅;苔黄厚,舌质红为病邪入里,病情较重,主气分热盛;邪入营分,可见舌绛;邪入血分,可见舌质深绛或紫暗,苔少或无苔;说明不同的舌象提示病位浅深不同。内伤杂病中,若脏腑功能失常,亦可反映于舌。一般舌尖红起芒刺,属心火亢盛;舌边红,多属肝胆有热;舌苔白而厚腻,多因脾失健运,湿邪内阻,如见于湿浊、痰饮等;舌中苔黄厚腻,多属脾胃湿热;舌体颤动,多为肝风内动;舌体喎斜,为中风或中风先兆等。

The changes of the location of disease can be reflected by tongue accordingly. The thickness or thinness of the coating and the changes of the tongue body can reflect the deep or shallow location, and the light or sever scale of the disease. Because viscera have their representative areas on tongue body, many reflect different pathological changes in viscera. So in general, the light and shallow disease may cause the changes of tongue coating, while the deep and sever disease may results in the changes of tongue coating and texture at the same time. For example, the thin white coating suggests that the disease is in its initial stage, the disease is located in shallow part and it is an exterior syndrome. But the thick, yellow coating and red tongue suggests that the disease is severe, and there is excessive heat in the *qi* phase, it is an interior syndrome. The crimson tongue indicates that the evils have entered into the *ying* phase. The deep crimson or dark purple tongue with little coating or without any coating means the evils into the blood phase. All of the above shows that the shallow or deep location of disease can be reflected by different changes of the tongue. The tongue also can reflect the abnormal function of viscera in diseases that are caused by internal injury. In general, prickles on the red tongue tip are due to flourishing heat evil in the heart, red color on the sides of tongue are due to heat in the liver and gallbladder. The white, thick and greasy coating mostly indicates that spleen fails to transport and transform nutrients and there is retention of dampness in the interior. It can be seen in diseases such as dampness-turbid and phlegm. The yellow, thick and greasy coating in the middle of the tongue is mostly due to damp-heat in spleen and stomach. The trembling tongue body often results from up stirring of the liver. The wry tongue body is usually a result of wind-stroke or an omen of wind-stroke.

4. 推断病势进退
4. To infer the Tendency of disease

通过对舌象的动态观察,可测知疾病发展的进退趋势。从舌苔上看,若苔色由白转黄,由黄转为灰黑,苔质由薄转厚,由润转燥,多为病邪由表入里,由轻变重,由寒化热,邪热内盛,津液耗伤,为病势发展。反之,若舌苔由厚变薄,由黄转白,由燥转润,为病邪渐退,津液复生,病情向好的方向转变。若舌苔骤增骤退,多为病情暴变所致。如薄苔突然增厚,是邪气急骤入里的表现;若满舌厚苔突然消退,是邪盛正衰,胃气暴绝的表现,二者皆为恶候。从舌质上看,舌色由淡红转为红、绛或绛紫,或舌面有芒刺、裂纹,是邪热内入营血,有伤阴、血瘀之势;若淡红舌转淡白、淡紫湿润,舌体胖嫩有齿痕,为阳气受伤,阴寒内盛,病邪由表入里,由轻转重,病情由单纯变为复杂,为病进。

The changes of tongue usually follow the changes of genuine *qi* and evils, and disease location, so we can infer the development and tendency of the disease by observing mobile changes of the tongue. For example, the turning of coating color from white to yellow, and from yellow to gray-black, and the turning of coating texture from thin to thick, or from moist to dry, is usually due to the transferring of evils from exterior to interior, or from light to sever, or from cold to heat, and the impairment and exhaustion of body fluid by the internal flourishing heat evils. It shows the deterioration of disease. On the contrary, the turning of coating color from yellow to white, and the coating texture from thick to thin, or from dry to moist, is mostly due to the slow withdrawal of evils and the new production of body fluid. It shows the recovery of disease. The sudden increasing or decreasing of coating usually results from the abrupt changes of disease. The immediate turning of coating from thin to thick is a sign of evils entering into the interior quickly. But the abrupt withdrawal from the thick coating on the whole tongue surface is due to excessive flourishing evils and deficient *vital-qi*, or violent exhaustion of *stomach-qi*. Both of them are serious signs. If the tongue color turns from pink to red, crimson or crimson purple, or there are prickles and fissure on the tongue surface, it suggests that the heat evils have entered into the *ying* and blood phase and have tendency to injure yin and result in blood stasis. If the tongue color turns from pink to pale, or pale purple, or there are teeth-prints on the margin of the fat, tender tongue body, it is due to the injured yang and the internal flourishing cold. It is a sign of that the evils have entered into the interior from the exterior and the turning of disease from light to sever. It shows the deterioration of disease.

5. 估计病情预后
5. To Estimate the Prognosis of Disease

舌荣有神,舌面有苔,舌态正常者,为邪气未盛,正气未伤,胃气未败,预后较好;舌质枯晦,舌苔无根,舌态异常者,为正气亏虚,胃气衰败,病情多凶险。

If the tongue vitality is vigorous and there is coating on the surface of the tongue, and the movement of the tongue is in normal, it is a condition that the evils is not flourishing, the *vital-qi* is not injured and the *stomach-qi* is not exhausted. It shows that the prognosis is good. The withering tongue texture with non-rooted coating and abnormal movement indicates the deficiency of *vital-qi* and the exhaustion of *stomach-qi*. It shows severity of the disease.

第二节 舌诊的临床应用
Section 2 Clinical Application of Tongue Inspection

舌象变化,随着病情的变化而变化,舌诊在诊治临床变化多端的疾病中,得到广泛应用,发挥着重要作用。

The changes of tongue pictures vary with changes of disease condition, tongue inspection is widely used and plays important role in diagnosing and treating the various disease.

1. 舌诊在温病诊治中的应用[1-5]

1. Application of tongue inspection in diagnosing and treating febrile disease$^{(1\sim5)}$

清代温病学家叶天士在《温热论》中,突出了舌诊在温病诊治中的重要作用和特殊的指导意义,首创卫气营血辨证。温病舌诊,临床主要从舌体的色泽、形态,舌苔的性状、颜色、润燥等方面来确定病位的浅深,辨别病邪的性质,区分证候的类型,判断津液的存亡,推断预后吉凶,为治疗提供依据。

Ye tianshi, a physician in Qing dynasty, stressed the important function and specially guiding significance and firstly created the syndrome differentiation of wei-qi-ying-xue. In his work *Treatise on Warm-heat*. Tongue inspection of febrile disease, clinically identify the evil nature, differentiate the types of syndromes, judge the depletion of fluid or not, make prognosis and offer foundation for treatment, from tongue body, shape and nature of tongue coating, color and luster, moistness and dryness.

(1) 辨舌苔探病邪性质、病位浅深

(1) To judge the nature of disease and to detect the location of disease

杜氏[1]认为温病在发生、发展过程中,虽然具有发病急骤、来势较猛、变化较多和病情较重等特点,但皆可通过舌质、舌苔的变化而显示出来。一般说来,温病舌苔的变化,随着苔色从浅变深,病情亦由浅向深重方向发展。苔色由白→黄→灰→黑,多为病邪由表入里,由轻变重,由浅入深。薄者较轻,厚者病重、润者津液未伤,燥者津液已伤。宋氏[2]等为继承和发扬叶天士的温病学说,研究了叶天士有关舌诊的论述,归纳为辨察舌苔,定卫气营血、定病机法方、定预后吉凶。刘氏[3]总结湿温病辨舌诊治经验时认为:舌苔厚腻是诊断湿温病的重要依据,但湿热秽浊之邪郁闭时,亦可见舌上仅有粘腻似苔非苔,并非都见厚腻。黄氏[4]等研究发现,舌苔黄厚而干,甚则焦黄起刺,为气分热结胃肠,苔黄燥焦黑,为热结阴伤。

Du[1] considered that during the course and development of febrile disease, It could be reflected through the changes of tongue texture and tongue coating, although febrile disease had characters of acute and dramatic onset and serious condition. Generally speaking, the more deeper the tongue color is , the more deeper and more critical the disease is . changes of coating color has a rule of white → yellow → gray →black , it means exogenous evils form exterior to interior ,the condition from slight to serious , from shallow to deep , if the coating is thin , it means slight condition, thick coating means serious condition, moistness means non-injured fluid, dryness means injured fluid. Song[2] concluded examining and differentiating tongue, located phrase of Wei-qi-yin-xue, made a method of mechanism and prognosis in order to develop and inherit the school of Ye Tianshi's febrile disease by researching the statements of Ye Tianshi. Liu[3] considered that thick and greasy coating was important basis for diagnosing the damp-warm disease when summing up the experience of differentiating damp-warm disease by tongue inspection, however, stick and greasy coating could be seen when the damp-heat and turbid evils were stagnated and obstructed. Huang[4] found out if the coating was thick and yellow with dryness, even brown with prickle, it indicated heat evils accumulated in gastrointestinal tract; if the coating is yellow ,dry, brown black, it suggested injured *yin* due to heat accumulation.

(2) 辨舌色定卫气营血、病情轻重
(2) To judge Wei-qi-yin-xue and the condition of disease

杜氏[1]认为温病如果舌苔的变化,演化为舌质的变化,多标志着病势的发展,病情更重,病位更深,多由卫气分深入营血分。在舌色方面,随着颜色的加深,热邪亦更加深入。红舌为初入营分,绛舌是热入营分之证,而紫舌是热入血分之证。张氏[5]研究了叶氏之论,认为舌质红绛是温病邪在营血的重要标志。营热则舌绛而干,动血则舌质紫绛。

Du[1] considered that if the changes of the coating evolved the changes of tongue texture, it mostly symbolized developments of the disease ,more serious condition and deeper location of disease, it meant that Wei-qi phrase entered Yin-xue phrase. As far as tongue color is concerned, the more color deepen, the more heat evils deepens into. Red tongue means initial Yin phrase, crimson tongue means syndrome of heat entering Yin phrase, however, purple tongue is syndrome of heat entering Xue phrase. Zhang[5] considered by researching the statements of Ye that crimson tongue is a important symbol of warm evil in Yin-Xue phrase. Tongue was crimson and dryness when heat in Yin phrase, tongue is purple and crimson when blood stirred.

2. 舌诊在心血管疾病诊治中的应用[6-12]
2. Application of tongue inspection in diagnosing and treating cardiovascular disease

祖国医学认为"心开窍于舌",舌与心在生理和病理方面有着密切联系,目前研究发现舌象的变化能及时灵敏地反映心血管的功能状态,对心血管疾病的诊断辨证、治疗预后等都有重要的指导意义。

T.C.M consider "the heart open into the tongue", they have close relationships with physiology and pathology. Recent researches found out that the changes of tongue picture can sensitively and promptly reflect the functional condition of the cardiovascular, and that have a guiding significance in treating and diagnosing and prognosis of cardiovascular diseases.

(1) 心肌梗死
(1) Myocardiacl infarction

高氏[6]对69例冠心病急性心肌梗死(AMI)患者进行了动态的观察,结果发现AMI的早期舌质红,苔黄燥,瘀热腑实证突出;在中期腻苔增多,舌质红紫,痰瘀壅阻为主证;而后期则为气阴两虚兼血瘀为主,舌质多呈暗红,舌苔薄白或无苔。张氏[7]对200例AMI患者进行了舌象分析,发现舌质淡红、舌质暗或紫暗辨证为气虚血瘀的共131例,占65.5%。

Gao[6] dynamically observed 69 AMI patients, and found out that in initial stage, tongue texture was red, coating was yellow and dry, which indicated blood stasis, heat and fu-visceral excess syndrome. In the middle stage, most of the patients' tongue were greasy, tongue textures were red and purple, which suggested the syndrome of phlegm-stasis retention; however, in late stage, most of the patients pertained to deficiency of both qi and yin accompanied with blood stasis, the tongue textures were dark red, the coatings were thin white or bare. Zhang[7] analyzed 200 tongue pictures on AMI patients, and found out that blood stasis cases whose tongue textures were reddish, dark or dark purple were 131, amounted to 65.5%.

AMI患者随病情的进展,舌苔变化迅速而明显。高氏[8]研究发现在AMI发病早期24小时之初舌苔主要为薄白或腻苔,薄白苔的发病率为41.3%,而随病情的进展则薄白苔逐渐降低,腻苔的出现率则增高,3天时黄腻苔和白腻苔上升为首位,以后随病情好转则腻苔减少,而薄白苔增多。总之,AMI的舌苔动态变化为薄→腻→薄、白→黄→白的演变规律,而净苔或剥苔随病情的进展趋于增多;舌质则红舌变化最剧,出现率由高到低递减,而暗红舌和紫舌则缓慢地稳步递增。

The tongue coatings changes rapidly with the development of diseases, Gao[8] found out initial stage (within 24 hours) of AMI patients most were thin white or greasy coating, and the accurate rate of thin white coating was 41.3%, however, the rate of thin white coating was decreased with the development of disease, the rate of greasy coating was increasing, yellow greasy coating ranked first in 3 days, with the development of improvement of diseases, greasy coating decreased, the thin white coating increased. In brief, dynamic changes of AMI was thin → greasy →thin, white→ yellow→ white, bare tongue and exfoliative tongue gradually increase with development of disease, In tongue texture, red tongue changed dramatically, the coincidences rate of it decreased from high to low, however, the dark red tongue and purple tongue increased gradually and steadily.

李氏[9]在陈旧性心肌梗死(OMI)的治疗上,依据舌象辨证处方,取得了很好的疗效。当舌质淡暗,或有瘀点瘀斑,提示气虚血瘀,治宜益气活血,通脉止痛,方用参芪逐瘀汤加减。舌淡紫,有瘀点瘀斑,苔白滑,提示阳虚血瘀,治宜温阳益气,活血通痹,方用温心汤加减。舌质暗,有瘀点瘀斑,苔腻,提示痰浊血瘀,治宜化瘀泄浊,活血化瘀,方用栝楼薤白散合血府逐瘀汤加减。苔白腻,提示痰湿壅盛,治宜健脾化痰,宣痹通阳,方用二陈汤加减。苔黄腻,提示痰热阻络,治宜清热化痰,行气止痛,方用血府逐瘀汤加减。舌质暗红,苔干或剥,提示气阴两虚夹瘀,治宜益气滋阴,活血化瘀,方用生脉散加减。

Li[9] prescribed formulas on the basis of tongue differentiation and curative effect was much improved in treating OMI. If tongue was dark pale, or with spots, it suggested qi deficiency and blood stasis, so it should be treated by strengthening the qi and activating blood circulation and promoting blood circulation and relieving pain. The formula was modified Shenqizhuyu decoction. If tongue was pale and purple with spots, the coating was white and slippery, it suggested yang deficiency and blood stasis, it should be treated by warming yang and strengthening the qi, removing obstruction and activating blood circulation, the formula was modified warming heart decoction. If tongue texture was dark with spots and greasy coating, it suggested turbid phlegm and blood stasis, and it should be treated by removing blood stasis and eliminating the turbid, activating blood circulation and removing blood stasis, the formula was gualou xie bai shan accompanied with xue fu zhu yu, If coating was greasy, it suggested phlegm-turbid accumulation, and should be treated by strengthening spleen and resolving phlegm, dispelling obstruction and promoting yang circulation, the formula is modified ercheng decoction. if coating was yellow greasy, and it suggested phlegm-heat obstructing the collaterals, and should be treated by clearing away heat and resolving phlegm, promoting qi circulation and relieving pain, formula is modified xuefuzhuyu decoction, If tongue is dark red, the coating was dry or exfoliate, it suggested deficiency of both qi and yin accompanied with blood stasis, and should be treated by strengthening qi and nourishing yin, activating blood circulation and removing blood stasis, the formula was modified shengmaisan

(2) 冠心病心绞痛

(2) Angina pectoris

一般的心绞痛患者,舌象可无明显的变化,但是若出现病理生理障碍时,则出现相应的舌象改变。冠心病辨证为气虚和阳虚的患者的主要舌象为淡白舌和胖嫩舌,这与冠心病患者左心功能减退是一致的;而冠心病血瘀证的主要舌象表现为青紫舌,这与冠心病患者的血液的改变是一致的。舌下静脉的改变与冠心病的发生亦密切相关。张氏[10]观察了100例缺血性心脑血管疾病的患者,发现舌下静脉扩张者内、中带均占100%,外侧带占78.51%;扭曲者内、中带平均占98.81%,外侧带占83.33%;瘀点者,内中平均占92.85%。

The tongue pictures has no obvious changes during moderate angina pectoris, however, if it occurs physiological or pathological obstacle, the tongue picture would change, the chief tongue picture are almost pale, corpulent, tender with differentiated qi deficiency and yang deficiency. This is consistent with the declination of left heart function; while the chief tongue pictures of coronary heart disease pertaining to blood stasis are blue and purple tongue, it also is consistent with the changes of blood circulation of coronary heart disease patients. Changes of vessels below tongue has close relationship with coronary heart disease, Zhang[10] observed 100 patients with ischemic cardiovascular and cerebrovascular diseases, and found out dilated vessels in internal and middle region amounted to 100%, external region 78.51%, distortedly internal and middle region 98.81%, external region 83.33%, in patients with spots, internal and middle region amounted to 92.85%.

(3) 房颤

(3) Atrial fibrillation

房颤是心律失常的一种类型,分为阵发型和持久型。叶氏[11]观察了两种房颤的舌象变化,发现两种房颤的舌象变化特点为:阵发型房颤病例中淡白舌所占比例大,持久型则舌质偏紫和暗红、胖大舌的比例则更大,因为阵发型房颤时左室射血功能减低,心排血量减少,而迟发型则多为阳虚血瘀故多偏紫和胖大。房颤的舌苔多为薄白苔,伴有心衰者,多兼有腻苔,说明心衰者有阳虚水泛或痰湿内停的病理,若舌苔增腻增厚往往并发他证而加重病情。

Atrial fibrillation is one kind of arrhythmia, and divided into paroxysmal and permanent type, Ye[11] observed the tongue picture changes of two kinds, and found out the character of two kinds : the percentage of pale tongue in paroxysmal atrial fibrillation was high, the percentage of purple, dark red, corpulent tongue in permanent atrial fibrillation is more higher, because ejection function of left cardiac ventricle and cardiac output decreased, however, most delayed type patients pertained to yang deficiency and blood stasis, so the tongue was purple and corpulent. The coating of atrial fibrillation is thin white coating, if accompanied with heart failure, it often is accompanied with greasy coat, which explains pathogenesis of yang deficiency and water insulting; If the coating became greasier and thicker than before , the disease become more serious because of accompanied other diseases.

3. 舌诊在肺系疾病诊治中的应用[12-15]
3. Application of tongue inspection in diagnosing and treating lung disease

舌诊在慢性支气管炎、肺心病、肺癌等疾病的诊治中具有重要的指导意义。
Tongue inspection has an important guiding significance in diagnosing and treating chronic bronchitis, pulmonary heart disease, and lung cancer.

(1) 慢性支气管炎、肺心病
(1) Chronic bronchitis , pulmonary heart disease

吴氏[12]认为舌质舌苔的变化情况可以用来判断慢性支气管炎、肺心病患者的病情程度,旧病是否新染,及是否夹有血瘀等。他认为慢性支气管炎、肺心病患者见舌质淡,苔薄白滑润者,是脾虚不运、水湿上溢、痰浊上犯所致;若舌质淡白偏暗,舌苔由白转黄,颗粒紧密胶结,是脾虚痰湿迁延日久化热、湿热痰涎胶结所致;若舌质淡红而胖大,舌面有小裂纹出现,舌苔洁白而碎腐、少津光亮,为脾阳衰败、寒湿凝闭、痰浊阻肺之候,多见于肺心病人的危重症;若肺心病患者的舌中间出现两条黄苔,干湿适中常提示肺心病合并感染;若舌质淡红边有成片青紫瘀斑,呈光剥样,或舌下静脉青黑怒张,舌质暗红者,多为血瘀。孙氏[13]依据舌象将肺心病患者分为四型,即痰热郁肺:舌质红、苔黄腻;痰湿蕴肺:舌质红、苔白腻;肺肾两虚:舌质绛、苔白腻或光剥;肺脾肾俱虚:舌质青暗而干、苔白腻或白滑。刘氏[14]对61例肺心病人的舌质进行了观察发现,在肺心病急性发作期,其舌质以红舌为主,共41例占67.2%;舌苔以腻苔为主,共32例占52.3%。

Wu[12] considered the changes of tongue texture and tongue coating can judge the condition of chronic bronchitis, pulmonary heart disease, and if there is new infection or not, with blood stasis or not. He considered that chronic bronchitis, pulmonary heart disease have pale tongue, slippery and thin white coating resulted from deficiency spleen failing to transport, water-dampness and turbid phlegm reverse attacking; If dark reddish tongue, the coating changed yellow from white, and fine particles was hard to scrapped, it resulted from spleen deficiency and prolonged phlegm-damp transforming into heat, and phlegm -heat-damp-saliva accumulation; If tongue is reddish and corpulent , and small crack was seen on the tongue surface , coating is white and broken putrid , little fluid and brightness, it was syndrome of depletion of spleen yang , coagulation and obstruction of damp-cold ,turbid phlegm obstructing lung , often seen in critical condition of pulmonary heart disease, If a yellow coating was seen on the tongue surface in pulmonary heart disease patients ,it indicated that patients suffered from pulmonary heart disease accompanied with infections. It indicated blood stasis when reddish tongue with blue spots and ecchymosis on both margins looking like exfoliation, or engorged blue vessels, dark red tongue were seen in clinic. Sun[13] divided pulmonary heart disease into four types based on tongue picture, e.g. stagnated phlegm-heat in lung: red tongue texture, yellow greasy coating; accumulated phlegm-dampness in lung, red tongue, white greasy coating; deficiency of both lung and kidney: crimson tongue, white greasy coating or exfoliation; deficiency of lung, spleen and kidney: dry and dark purple, white greasy and white slippery coating. Liu[14] observed 61 pulmonary heart disease cases on tongue texture, and found out that in acute attack of pulmonary heart disease, patients predominantly having red tongue were 41, amounting to 67.2%, patients predominantly having greasy coating were 32, amounting to 52.3%.

(2) 肺癌
(2) Lung cancer

苏氏[15]通对380例原发性肺癌患者舌象进行观察分析,发现舌象对肺癌分期有一定的参考价值。舌质淡红、舌苔薄而质润,多为病之早期;舌质红或紫、舌苔厚而腐腻,多为肺癌中晚期。本组病例紫舌213例,占56.05%。舌质由紫转淡红或晦暗转明润,舌苔由厚变薄,由无苔变薄苔,说明病情好转,反之为逆;舌红绛少苔或无苔表示胃气已绝,预后差。舌诊可预测患者对放疗的耐受性,可供确定放射治疗剂量时的参考,还可指导治疗用药。

Su[15] observed and analyzed 380 tongue pictures suffering from primary lung cancer, found out that tongue pictures offered certain value for dividing stages of lung cancer. If seen reddish tongue, thin and moist coating, we can infer it as early stage, If seen red or purple tongue and thick and putrid coating, we can infer it as middle or late stage. Patients with purple tongue in this group were 213, amount to 56.05%. It suggests improvement of disease when purple tongue change from reddish or dim tongue changed to brightness, coating changed from thick to thin, or from bare to thin. On the contrary, is called deterioration; If tongue was red crimson with little coating or without coating, it suggested depletion of stomach qi, the prognosis was unfavorable. Tongue inspection can predict the tolerance of radioactivity to patients and offer reference for dosage of radioactivity, guide treatment and drug-use as well.

4. 舌诊在脾胃疾病诊治中的应用[16-23]
4. Application of tongue inspection in diagnosing and treating spleen and stomach disease

"舌为脾胃的外候",舌象的改变与脾胃疾病密切相关,不同病理类型胃炎及溃疡患者的舌象各有不同的特点。

"Tongue is called the out-show of the spleen and stomach", changes of tongue pictures has a close relationship with spleen and stomach disease, tongue picture has different characters matching different types of gastritis and peptic ulcer.

(1) 慢性胃炎
(1) Chronic gastritis

幽门螺杆菌(HP)与舌苔有着密切的关系。近年来国内外学者普遍认为慢性胃炎与HP的感染有关,魏氏[16]等观察了有HP感染的胃炎患者的舌苔,结果发现两者之间有一定关系,即有HP感染的患者多为白腻苔、黄腻苔或黄苔。HP开始侵袭胃粘膜,出现湿困脾阳,舌苔以白腻苔为主;久之化热,而出现黄腻苔或黄苔。HP的感染与舌质无关。

Hp has close relationship with coating, Recently the scholars in domestic and abroad widely considered that chronic gastritis has relationship with infection of Hp, Wei[16] observed the coating with Hp infected gastritis, found out both had certain relation, e.g. the coating of patients with Hp infection were white greasy coating, yellow greasy coating or yellow coating. It occurred inspleen yang encumbered by dampness, and the coating will be white greasy coating when Hp invade the gastric mucosa, If Hp infection is no completely eradicated for long time, it will be transforming into heat, and then the yellow greasy coating or yellow coating will occur. The Hp infection has nothing to do with tongue texture.

胃炎的病理程度不同,舌质和舌苔亦出现相应的变化。何氏[17]研究发现慢性浅表性胃炎的舌苔多黄或厚,慢性萎缩性胃炎的舌苔多为正常,慢性浅表性萎缩性胃炎的舌苔以黄厚苔为多,并发现在治疗过程中消退较慢。并提出黄苔的形成可能与胃内的炎症有关。陈氏[18]观察发现浅表性胃炎病程较短,淡红舌所占的比例较萎缩性胃炎及其伴肠化生者大,而后者青紫舌所占的比重大,常被认为是癌前病变。丁氏[19]观察发现慢性萎缩性胃炎病人中,舌质红,少津无苔,胃阴虚型者占60%,所以在治疗中慎用香燥辛热之品。

Tongue texture and tongue coating will correspond with the pathologic extent of gastritis. He[17] found out that most tongue coatings of chronic superficial gastritis patients were yellow or thick, most tongue coatings of chronic atrophy gastritis were yellow thick coating, and inflammation faded gradually when treated. He proposed that the formation of yellow coating probably has something to do with gastric inflammation. Cheng[18] found out that the course of superficial gastritis is short, percentage of reddish tongue is higher than those of atrophy gastritis and atrophy gastritis accompanied with epithelial metaplasis, however, the percentage of blue tongue in the latter is higher, and considered as precancerous lesion. Ding[19] found out that in chronic atrophy gastritis, deficiency of stomach yin type whose tongue is red, little fluid without coating amounted to 60%, one should be cautious when using drugs whose nature pertain to pungent, dry and hot.

(2) 胃及十二指肠溃疡
(2) Gastric ulcer and duodenalulcer

何氏[20]认为溃疡活动期多有黄苔或厚苔,近愈者舌苔可正常,若合并慢性浅表性胃炎者均为黄厚苔。十二指肠溃疡的舌苔多无改变,只有当合并浅表性胃炎或胃溃疡时才有明显的改变。舌苔的变化对判断上述胃病的病情变化有一定价值。舌苔由厚变薄,由黄变白是好转的趋势,反之则加重。但是胃内病变程度相似的患者舌苔厚薄黄白的程度可以存在个体差异,尤其男女之间差别较明显。同一病人的舌苔进退就有很大的临床参考价值。舌象的变化可以帮助判断是否有穿孔,以及协助诊断穿孔的部位和性质。王氏[21]研究发现胃穿孔舌尖红绛光亮区范围增大,十二指肠穿孔舌尖红绛光亮区范围小。单纯性胃十二指肠穿孔舌色多见淡红、红或绛;而胃癌穿孔或伴消化道出血则舌质多青紫或淡白。舌质淡红者穿孔多小于0.5cm,腹腔渗液量多小于300ml;而红绛紫舌者穿孔多大于0.5cm,渗液量大于300ml;胃十二指肠穿孔时舌苔白则提示梗阻程度轻,黄苔或黑苔则重。

He[20] considered that in active ulcer stage most tongues were yellow coating or thick coating, the coating would be normal when the ulcer is cured, yellow thick coating would be seen when accompanied with chronic superficial gastritis, the tongue often had no changes in duodenal ulcer, only if accompanied with superficial gastritis or gastric ulcer, there would be obvious changes, so changes of tongue offer a certain value in judging gastric disease mentioned above. Coating changed from thick to thin, from yellow to white is a tendency of improvement. Vice versus, but patients who have similar degree pathologic changes may have significant differences, Especially between male and female. The tendency of tongue of same person has great reference value, changes of tongue picture can help us judge perforation or not, and help us diagnose the location and nature of perforation. Wang[21] found the area of crimson region on tongue tip would enlarge with existing gastric perforation, and the area of crimson region on tongue tip decrease with existing duodenal perforation. Most tongue color of simple gastric and duodenal perforation were reddish, red or crimson; however, most tongue were blue purple or pale when existing cancer perforation or hemorrhage of digestive tract. If tongue was reddish, the width of perforation was less than 0.5cm, and exudative hydrops was less than 300ml, if tongue was red, crimson and purple, the perforation was bigger than 0.5cm, exudative hydrops was more than 300ml, and white coating suggests mild obstruction with gastric and duodenal perforation. However, yellow coating or black coating suggests a severe condition.

(3) 急性阑尾炎
(3) Acute appendicitis

杨氏[22]观察发现急性阑尾炎的舌象有一定的变化规律,即舌面起红刺,色泽鲜明,分布与舌尖及其两侧,多为红刺粗大,舌苔多白滑或黄腻,常见于阑尾穿孔或化脓、坏疽;单纯性阑尾炎以薄白苔为主。经统计,应用舌象诊断,术前和术后的符合率达93.5%。王氏[23]观察发现不同病理类型的急性阑尾炎的舌象变化规律不同,即在舌尖变化的基础上,有白苔或薄黄苔出现;当阑尾为化脓性炎症时,就会增加舌质红或绛,并会出现厚腻苔;当阑尾坏疽时,不但舌尖、舌色、舌苔发生改变,还会出现瘀斑、瘀点;当阑尾穿孔发生腹膜炎时,舌尖红赤范围增宽,严重时舌面还出现亮光;若腹膜炎迁延不愈,舌苔之白腻黄腻苔还可出现剥脱现象;当水电解质发生紊乱,除原有舌色加深外,舌面常显示干燥或裂纹,舌中心苔焦黄或焦黑。

Yang[22] found out that tongue pictures of acute appendicitis had a certain rule, when existing appendix perforation or suppuration, gangrene, most tongue were white slippery or yellow greasy, most of patients have a thin white coating in simple appendicitis, it was statistically analyzed that the coincidence of preoperation and past operation is 93.5%. Wang[23] found out that different pathologic types of acute appendicitis had different rules of changing tongue. That is to say, on the basis of a white or thin yellow coating on tongue tip, tongue texture will become red or crimson when the nature of appendicitis is suppuration, and a thick greasy coating is seen. Not only will the tongue tip, tongue color and coating change, but also the ecchymosis or spots occur when there is existing gangrene, the red region of tongue would enlarge when appendicitis accompanies peritonitis, in severe case, brightness appears; If peritonitis was prolonged and not cured, white greasy, yellow greasy coating would be exfoliation, tongue surface will be cracked or dry, and there would be brown yellow or brown black in the middle of the tongue, except that the original color deepened, with existing water-electrolyte imbalance.

5. 舌诊在肝胆疾病诊治中的应用[24-29]

5. Application of tongue inspection in diagnosing and treating liver and gallbladder disease

近代研究发现舌与乙型肝炎病毒的感染有一定的联系,可以依据其特点判断肝胆疾病的感染情况,指导治疗及判断预后。肝硬化疾病的舌质、舌苔变化,能够反映出肝硬化在不同时期疾病轻重和进退。

Recent research has found out that the tongue has a certain relationship with infection HBV, and on the basis of its character, we can judge infection of liver and gallbladder disease, guide treatment, and judge prognosis, changes of tongue texture, coating can reflect the tendency and condition of different phase of the disease.

(1) 乙型肝炎及肝癌
(1) B hepatitis and liver cancer

张氏[24]对慢性乙型肝炎患者的舌象与病理进行了观察,结果发现慢性迁延性肝炎(CPH)舌质多无改变,为淡红舌,病理组织学以纤维组织增生,肝细胞松亮为主;慢性活动性肝炎(CAH)多为红舌或紫暗、瘀斑舌,舌为红色时,病理组织学以碎屑坏死、界板坏死、灶性坏死为主。慢性肝炎时舌苔的变化无太大的意义。以上观察结果与骆氏[25]的观察结果基本一致。骆氏认为CAH多为紫暗舌或瘀斑舌,提示瘀血阻络,治疗以滋阴疏肝的同时加用活血化瘀之品;CPH多为淡红舌,治疗以清热解毒为主。夏氏[26]观察发现,无症状的乙肝病毒携带者的舌象多为正常,说明邪气较轻,舌质持续为紫暗或有瘀斑,常提示病毒复制活跃,应及早加用活血化瘀之品,以防肝硬化发生。赵氏[27]提出治疗乙肝以舌诊为依据,辨证指导用药与变化剂量,并根据舌象的变化确定用药时间及调整方药。如乙肝患者舌质淡胖苔白腻,为脾虚湿困,应重用健脾化湿药,若舌苔转为正常,则化湿药减量,以免伤阴,此时应重用扶正解毒药。李氏[28]观察发现早期肝硬化多见舌质暗红,舌体较胖或边有齿痕;肝硬化代偿期,舌质青紫,舌上有青紫瘀斑;肝功能失代偿期腹水轻者,多见舌淡红,苔白腻;肝硬化后期,舌质紫红有瘀点、瘀斑,舌下静脉怒张,舌苔薄黄腻。

Zhang[24] observed tongue and pathology of chronic B hepatitis patients and found out that there were no obvious changes in the tongue which was a reddish tongue, there existed fibroplastic proliferation, the liver cells were loose and bright, In chronic hepatitis most tongues were red or dark purple or ecchymosis, when tongue was red, there mainly existed fragment necrosis, borderline necrosis, focal necrosis. Changes of tongue in chronic hepatitis had obvious significance, the results mentioned above was basically the same as those of Lo's, Lo[25] considered tongue of CAH mostly to be dark purple or ecchymosis tongue, which suggested blood stasis obstructed collaterals, so its therapy should be nourish Yin and disperse liver qi and add drugs activating blood circulation and removing the blood stasis, Tongue of CPH are mostly reddish, so the therapy should be clearing away the heat and toxin materials. Xia[26] has found out the tongue pictures of asymptomatic pathogenic virus carriers are normal, which suggest mild evils, If tongues are continuous dark purple or with eccchymosis, it suggests virus replication is active, drugs whose nature are activate blood circulation and remove blood stasis should be added in order to prevent the cirrhosis of liver. Zhao[27] proposed that drug-use, dosage, time of drug-use and regulation of drugs should be on basis of tongue inspection, If tongues of hepatitis B patients are pale, corpulent, coatings are white greasy, it indicates deficient spleen encumbered by dampness, and drugs strengthening spleen and resolving dampness should be used, If tongues and coatings change into normal, the dosages of resolving dampness drugs should decrease lest injure yin, on this occasion, High-dosage drugs strengthening the body resistance and clearing away toxins should be used, Li[28] has found out that dark red tongues, corpulent tongue body or teeth-print on both margins are often seen in early stage of cirrhosis of liver, In compensatory phase, bluish purple tongue and bluish purple ecchymosis are often seen in clinic, In decompensatory phase with less ascites, reddish tongues and white greasy coatings are often seen, in late stage of liver cirrhosis, there are reddish purple tongue with ecchymosis or spots, engorgedly blue vessels and thin, yellow, greasy coating.

(2) 胆囊炎、胆结石
(2) Cholecystitis, Cholelithiasis

李氏[28]通过对69例急性胆囊炎观察,发现患者舌苔以黄腻为主,少数为白腻苔,舌质多红,尤以舌边舌尖为著。说明急性胆囊炎主要由肝胆气滞、中焦湿热内阻所致。林氏[29]等报道苔薄白提示胆囊炎为慢性;舌色红或绛,舌边着色重则多提示胆囊炎为急性,有条纹者证明炎症是反复发生的,瘀斑点提示结石或炎症重。

LI[28] has observed 69 acute cholecystitis patients and found out that coatings mostly were yellow greasy , some were white greasy , tongue most were red especially on both margins and tongue tip, which suggested acute cholecystitis resulted from stagnation of liver and gallbladder qi , damp-heat accumulation in middle-Jiao. Ling[29] has reported that thin white coating suggested chronic cholecystitis , that crimson or red tongue ,deep color on tongue margin suggested acute cholecystitis, that cracks indicate recurrent inflammation ,that spots or ecchymosis indicated gallstone and severe inflammation .

6. 舌诊在肾脏疾病诊治中的应用[30-31]
6. Application of tongue inspection in diagnosing and treating kidney disease

在肾病范围内对舌象的诊察重点应注重舌色、荣嫩、齿印及印下色,舌苔厚薄的变化。大多数肾病的机体内环境尚稳定[30-31],舌象以正常淡红色为主,表现体内气血尚充。而当肾功能衰减时则淡白舌的出现率增加,此种舌象亦与水肿及贫血有一定的关联性。在动态观察中仅贫血一个因素较重时也会出现淡白舌,但也有血红蛋白虽低而舌色不变者;另一方面,有的血红蛋白不低,肾生化指标正常者出现淡白舌,在随后的观察中出现肾功能衰竭的表现,提示肾病出现淡舌应引起高度警惕与重视。

In kidney diseases, Attention should bepaid on tongue color, tender and tough, teeth-print , color below teeth-print,; most organism environments are stable(30-31). Reddish tongues suggest ample qi and blood. Incidence of pale tongue increases when kidney function decline, this kind of tongue picture also has certain relationship with edema and anemia. In dynamic observation, pale tongue may occur in severe anemia , but sometime the tongue color would not change even if low hematochrome, on other hand , pale tongue may occur even if hematochrome is not low and biochemical criterion of kidney are normal, It suggest doctors should keep alert and pay attention when pale tongue occur in kidney diseases in the following observation ,especially failure of kidney function occur,

慢性肾衰(CRF)的病理舌象主要表现为舌体胖大、有齿痕,舌体胖嫩,主要因血浆蛋白低下,全血黏度及血浆黏度降低所致。齿印舌的形成,主要是由于舌组织水肿而舌体胖大,压迫于齿龈上显出了齿印。亦有部分患者有不同程度的舌质淡紫、暗红、暗紫、瘀斑等瘀血的表现,主要是由于脾肾阳虚无力运血而致血脉瘀阻。CRF舌面津液测定值明显低于健康人组,说明CRF病变与舌面津液的变化有一定的联系。急性肾炎与肾病综合征急性期则表现为舌色过红,但是此期为正盛邪实,一时尚无大碍。CRF 舌苔以薄白苔,薄白腻苔为主,脾肾阳虚患者表现最为突出。舌苔的颜色在肾病中的诊断价值尚需进一步观察,因为在肾病的发展过程中舌色经常黄白相互转化,黄苔主热而白苔主寒的理论似乎不太适用。舌边横纹的变浅、变平、模糊不清、消失多提示肾功能不良。

Pathologic tongue pictures of CRF are mostly corpulent tongue body, teeth-print, corpulent tongue body that results from low hemoglobin and low blood viscosity, formation of teeth-print result from corpulent tongue body compressed by gums, some patient have different extent blood stasis manifestation such as purplish, dark red, dark purple, ecchymosis tongue, which mainly are due to yang deficiency of both spleen and kidney failing to transport blood and leads to obstruction of blood and vessels. Measurements of conductance of tongue fluid in CRF are obvious less than the healthy people, which suggest pathologic changes of CRF has certain relationship with tongue fluid. Manifestations of acute nephritis and nephrotic syndrome are red tongue, but in this phase its nature is prosperity of genuine-qi and evil-qi, which does not matter. Tongue of CRF are mainly thin white coating, thin white greasy coating, especially in yang deficiency of both spleen and kidney, the diagnostic value of tongue color on kidney diseases is not certain and needs further observation. The theory of yellow coating suggesting heat syndrome and white coating suggesting cold syndrome seems not applicable because yellow and white coating often change into each other in the development of kidney diseases. Transverse crack on margins becoming shallower, flatter, vague or disappearing often suggests kidney function in bad condition.

7. 舌诊在内分泌疾病诊治中的应用[32-34]
7. Application of tongue in diagnosing and treating endocrinopathy

近十几年的研究表明,舌与内分泌的关系并不仅仅是与舌面局部的相关因素有关,舌象变化还能反映机体的内分泌状态,许多内分泌疾病在舌上有特异性变化。淡白舌的形成与肾上腺皮质功能不足关系密切,但是光红舌质与甲状腺功能亢进有一定联系,激素是维持人体内外平衡的一个重要调节因素,对物质代谢有十分重要的影响。

Recently more than 10years researches suggest that the relationship between tongue and endocrinopathy have not only something to do with relevant factors of local tongue, but also the tongue picture can reflect the conditions of endocrine, plenty of endocrinopathies have specific changes on tongue. Formation of pale tongue has close relationship with adrenocortical insufficiency, however, bare red tongue has certain relationship with hyperparthyroidism

舌诊对糖尿病的辨治具有特别重要的意义。糖尿病因阴亏燥热而发病,且病程长,内伤重,涉及多个脏腑,导致气血津液阴阳的严重病变,舌象恰能及时反映其病变,为其立法施治提供依据。如患者舌质红而鲜艳,甚至尖有芒刺,苔薄而干者,宜清热养阴,生津止渴为治疗大法；舌质红而暗乏津，无苔或少苔者宜滋养肝肾、润燥止渴为主；舌质淡嫩，边有齿痕者以健脾益气、助运生津为治疗大法。周氏在临床中观察发现糖尿病患者的舌下络脉多迂曲、紫暗，提示有瘀血，其瘀血程度与病情、并发症有关，在治疗中应加以重视，并注意活血化瘀在本病中的运用。

  Tongue inspection offers very important significance on differentiation and treatment of diabetes. Diabetes leads to severe pathologic changes of qi-xue-body fluid because diabetes has a long course, severe injure and involves many zang and fu viscera and result from yin deficiency and dry-heat. Tongue pictures can promptly reflect its pathologic changes, and offer a basis for therapeutic principle and treatment, for example, doctors should clear away heat and nourish yin, promote production of body fluid and quench thirst if seeing red and fresh tongue even prickle, dry and thin coating; if seeing dark red and less fluid tongue, no coating or less coating, the principle of nourishing liver and kidney, moistening dryness and quenching thirst should be adopted, if seeing tender tongue with teeth-print on both margins, doctors should strengthen spleen, replenish qi and promote production of body fluid. Zhou has found out in clinic observations that diabetes patients have dark purple, curved vessels below tongue which suggest blood stasis, the extent of blood stasis has something to do with conditions and complications, so doctors should pay attention to it and application of drugs of activating blood circulation and removing blood stasis.

参 考 文 献
Reference documents

[1] 杜松松．略论温病之舌诊．湖北中医杂志，1992，14(5)：30-31
Du songsong, simple exposition on tongue inspection of warm disease. Hubei journal of traditional Chinese Medicine 1992,14(5):30-31

[2] 宋文海，等．叶天士舌诊探析．江西中医学院学报，1993，5(1)：21-22
Song wenhai,etal discussion and analysis on ye tianshi tongue inspection Acta Academiae Medicinae Jiangxi 1993,5(1):21-22

[3] 刘继智．湿温辨舌临床体会．实用中医药杂志，1993，(1)29-30
Liu jizhi. Clinic experience on tongue differentiation of warm-dampness Journal of Practical Traditional Chinese Medicine 1993.(1):29-30

[4] 张炳立．叶天士论绛舌证治．天津中医，1996，(2)：6-7
Zhang bingli expostition on syndrome and treatment of crimson by ye tianshi Tianjin Journal of Traditional Chinese Medicine 1996.(2):6-7

[5] 黄淑方，等．舌诊在温病通下泄热治疗中的应用．中国医刊，1999，34(12)：43-44
Huang shufang etal, tongue inspection application of purgation and expelling heat Chinese Journal of Medicine 1999,34(12):43-44

[6] 高秀梅，等．急性心肌梗死舌象的动态观察及实验研究．天津中医，1980，8(10)：634
Gao xiumei etal, dynamic observation and experimental research on AMI Tianjin Journal of Traditional Chinese Medicine 1980.8(10):634

[7] 张九山等．肺心病患者舌质的临床与实验观察．天津中医，1980，8(4)：206〗
Zhang jiushan etal, clinic and experimental observation on tongue of pulmonary heart disease Tianjin journal of Traditional Chinese Medicine 1980,8(4):206

[8] 高秀梅．急性心肌梗死的特殊舌象．中医杂志，1994，35(3)：365
Gao xiumei special tongue pictures of AMI Journal of T.C.M 1994;35(3):365

[9] 李春杰．辨证治疗陈旧性心肌梗死 30 例观察．中医函授通讯，2000,19(3)：22-24
LiI chunjie ,differentiation and treatment on 30 case of OMI T.C.M Journal of correspondent communication 2000,19(3):22-24

[10] 张华一．"舌脉"预测冠心病、脑中风的研究．实用中西医结合杂志，1993，6(6)：389
Zhang huayi tongue predicting coronary heart disease and windstroke Journal of practical T.C.M and west Medicine 1993.6(6):389

[11] 叶仰光．88 例老年慢性房颤的舌象观察．福建中医药，1992，23(2)：31-32
Ye yangguang tongue observation on 88 case of aged chronic Atrial fibrillation Fujiang Journal of T.C,M 1992.23(2):31-32

[12] 吴济川．浅谈舌诊在慢性支气管炎、肺心病诊治中的应用．湖北中医杂志，2000,22(12).-19-19

Wu jichuan．simple exposition on tongue's application of diagnosing and treating chronic bronchitis and pulmonary heart diseases Hubei Journal of T.C.M 2000,22(12):19

[13] 孙洁民．肺心病舌象变化分型及病情预后判断．现代中西医结合杂志，2000，28(1)：38-38
Sun jiemin types and prognosis of tongue changes of pulmonary heart disease current journal of T.C.M and West Medicine 2000,28(1):38

[14] 刘建雯．61例肺心病病人舌象的临床观察．天津中医，1992,(2).-38-38,44
Liu jianwen tongue observation on 61 pulmonary heart disease patients Tianjin Journal of Traditional Chinese Medicine 1992,(2):38,34

[15] 苏晋梅．原发性肺癌380例舌象分析．山西中医，2000,16(5)：12-13
Su jingmei tongue analysis on 30 primary lung cancer Shanxi Journal of T.C.M 2000,16(5):12-13

[16] 魏学琴．张泉等．幽门螺杆菌与慢性胃炎的舌质、舌苔关系的分析．四川中医，1999,17(11)：7-8
Wei xueqin zhang qun etal．Analysis on Hp relationship with tongue and coating of chronic gastritis Shichuan Journal of T.C.M 1999,17(11):7-8

[17] 何晋森．，刘宇，等．溃疡病与慢性胃炎的舌苔观察．天津中医，2000,17(5)：16-17
He jinsen, Liu yu etal．Tongue observation on peptic ulcer and chronic gastritis Tianjin Journal of Traditional Chinese Medicine 2000,17(15):16-17

[18] 陈分乔．900例慢性萎缩性胃炎舌质与胃镜、病理相关性观察．河北中医，1999,21(11)：349-350
Cheng fengqiao, relevant observation on gastroscope and pathology with tongue of 900 chronic gastritis patients Hebei Journal of T.C.M 1999,21(11):349-350

[19] 丁创业．慢性萎缩性胃炎病人的中医舌诊浅析．实用中西医结合杂志．1996,9(2)：111-111
Ding chuangye simply analysis on tongue of chronic gastritis Journal of practical T.C.M and west Medicine 1996,9(2):111

[20] 何晋森,刘宇等．溃疡病与慢性胃炎的舌苔观察．天津中医，2000,17(5)：16-17
He jinsen, liuyu etal tongue observation on peptic ulcer and chronic gastritis Tianjin Journal of T.C.M

[21] 王淑英,张永丰等．变舌在十二指肠穿孔诊断中的价值．浙江中医杂志，1993,5：235-236
Wang shuying,zhang yong fong etal, value of changing tongue on diagnosing duodenal perforation Zhejiang Journal of T.C.M 1993(5):235-236

[22] 杨依芳．阑尾炎舌诊标志探索．中西医结合杂志，1984,(7)：398
Yang yifang symbolic tongue exploration on appendicitis journal of T.C.M combining West Medicine 1984,(7):398

[23] 王淑英,张永丰,等．489例急性阑尾炎患者舌象的分析．浙江中医杂志，1999,(9)：396
Wang shuying zhang yongfen,etal, tongue analysis on 489 acute appendicitis patients Zhejiang Journal of T.C.M 1999,(9):396

[24] 张赤志．对慢性乙型肝炎舌象与病理组织的观察．中国医药学报，1997,12(3)：44-44
Zhang chizhi histopathology observation with tongue picture of chronic B hepatitis China Journal of T.C.M 1997,12(3):44

[25] 骆群．慢性乙型肝炎患者舌象变化与肝脏病理学改变的关系．浙江中医学院学报，1996,20(5)：29-29
luo qun relationship between changing tongue picture of chronic B hepatitis patients and changes

of liver pathology journal of zhejiang college of T. C. M 1996,20(5):29

[26] 夏军权．乙型肝炎与无症状病毒携带者 295 例舌象观察．辽宁中医杂志，1995,22(7)：310-311
Xia junquan tongue observation between B hepatitis and 295 asymptomatic pathogenic virus carrier Liaoningli Journal of T. C. M 1995,22(7):310-311

[27] 赵兰稳．舌诊在乙型病毒性肝炎诊治过程中作用初探．河北中医,1999,21(5)：2900-290
Zhao lanwen simple exploration rule of tongue inspection on diagnosing and treating B hepatitis Hebei Journal of T. C. M 1999,21(5):190

[28] 李乃民．中医舌诊大全．北京:学苑出版社,1000-1319
Li naimin encycolopaedia of china tongue inspection Beijing academy press 1000-1039

[29] 林宗广．急性胆囊炎 69 例临床分析与病机、治疗初探．中医杂志,1964,(3)：1-4
Ling zhongguan clinic analysis and pathogenesis and treatment exploration on 69 acute cholecystitis Journal of T. C. M 1964,(3):1-4

[30] 杜家和．137 例肾病舌象的动态观察．中国中医基础杂志,2002,8(8)：39-40
Du jiahe dynamically tongue observation on 137 kidney diseases 2002,8(8):39-40

[31] 宋金海．慢性肾衰的舌诊研究．天津中医,1992,(6)：34-36
Song jinghai tongue inspection research on CRF Tianjin journal of T. C. M 1992,(6):；34-36

[32] 李灿东．中医舌诊与内分泌相关性研究的进展．福建中医学院学报,2001,11(2)：58-60
Li changdong relevant development on endocrine and tongue inspection Fujiang Journal of T. C. M 2001,11(2)：58-60

[33] 田志高．舌诊对糖尿病辨治的指导意义．北京中医,1997,(2)：9
Tian zhigao guiding significance of tongue inspection on syndrome differentiation of diabetes Beijing Journal of T. C. M 1997,(2)：9

[34] 周建扬．舌底络脉瘀血与糖尿病．浙江中医杂志,2000,35(2)：88
Zhou jiangyang blood stasis of vessels below tongue and diabetes Zhejiang Journal of T. C. M 2000,35(2):88

图书在版编目（CIP）数据

中医舌诊图谱(中英文对照)/丁成华等主编.—北京：
人民卫生出版社,2003
　ISBN 7-117-05767-X

　Ⅰ.中… Ⅱ.丁… Ⅲ.舌诊－图谱
Ⅳ.R241.25-64

中国版本图书馆 CIP 数据核字(2003)第 092846 号

中 医 舌 诊 图 谱
（中英文对照）

主　　编：丁成华　孙晓刚
出版发行：人民卫生出版社(中继线 67616688)
地　　址：(100078)北京市丰台区方庄芳群园 3 区 3 号楼
网　　址：http://www.pmph.com
E - mail：pmph@pmph.com
印　　刷：北京人卫印刷厂(尚艺)
经　　销：新华书店
开　　本：787×1092　1/16　印张：8.5
字　　数：182 千字
版　　次：2003 年 12 月第 1 版　2005 年 1 月第 1 版第 2 次印刷
标准书号：ISBN 7-117-05767-X/R·5768
定　　价：41.00 元

著作权所有，请勿擅自用本书制作各类出版物，违者必究
（凡属质量问题请与本社发行部联系退换）